The ART of Being Healthy

Volume 1

The ART of Being Healthy

Wellness Concepts From the Pros

Dr. Dustin Barton
Dr. Natalie Bird
Dr. Jessica Dietrich-Marsh
Dr. Ryan French
Dr. Robert Kipp
Dr. Michelle Krenek
Dr. Gilles LaMarche
Dr. Todd Lizon
Dr. Kunal Patel
Dr. Larisa Shevchuk
Dr. Bettina Tornatora
Dr. Devin Vrana
Dr. Krysti Wick

ISBN: 978-0-9898430-0-3

Library of Congress Control Number: 2013914965

Printed and bound in the United States of America

Cover & Text Design by www.tothepointsolutions.com

This book is dedicated to everyone who has contributed to telling the truth about health and healing; to the professionals and other ambassadors who endeavor to carry these messages forward; to the students enrolled in Chiropractic schools around the world; and to all people, children and adults alike, who will benefit from the wisdom shared herein.

A very special thank you to Jeff Hays and Bobby Sheehan, Producer and Director of the critically acclaimed documentary Doctored. *We sincerely appreciate your commitment to exposing the truth in search of better health naturally.*

CONTENTS

The five most dangerous words in the English language:

Maybe it will go away.

PREFACE

Dr. Gilles LaMarche

The most precious gift in life is your health. If you don't believe me, ask anyone who is chronically ill and/or fighting a disease what they want most, and they will tell you without hesitation "my health."

The World Health Organization (WHO) describes *health* as follows: "Health is a state of complete physical, mental and social well-being and not merely the absence of disease or infirmity." This definition has not been altered since 1948, and yet, what we might call modern society has come to recognize health as being "the absence of symptoms and disease."[1]

Due to the quick-fix theory that so many live by, people think that the answer to all ailments can be found in the utilization of a drug or chemical. Rather than looking for the cause of health, science has concentrated on trying to find the cause of disease, and on defining the ability to fight disease. Traditional medicine works at eliminating or controlling signs and symptoms of a disease that has invaded an individual by utilizing chemical means or external invasive forces, such as surgery. It is mechanistic in nature, uses drugs to resist death, attempts to control the variables, and battles the disease by attempting to take over the body's wisdom while working at relieving pain and postponing death.

Yet, this is not health.

The dedication of the majority of medical doctors is without doubt; the wonderful advancements that have taken place regarding crisis-care in medicine are obvious—and for that we are grateful. Yet, at the same time, there have been major abuses of power. The fact that pharmaceutical companies want to control everything that is perceived as health or health care is definitely a concern.

In the book *The Truth About Drug Companies*, it says: "Drug companies are involved in every detail of research, from design of the study through analysis of the data, to decision whether to publish the results or not. That involvement has made bias not only possible

---

1. Preamble to the Constitution of the World Health Organization as adopted by the International Health Conference, New York, 19-22 June, 1946; signed on 22 July 1946 by the representatives of 61 States (Official Records of the World Health Organization, no. 2, p. 100) and entered into force on 7 April 1948

but also extremely likely. Researchers don't control clinical trials anymore, sponsors do."[2] In his book *Over-Diagnosed: Making People Sick in the Pursuit of Health*, Dr. H. Gilbert Welch provides information regarding changes made to what is considered normal test values. For example, in the past, if you had a fasting blood sugar over 140, you had diabetes. In 1997, The Expert Committee on the Diagnoses of Diabetes Mellitus redefined the disorder. Now, if you have a fasting blood sugar over 126 you have diabetes. That little change from 140 to 126 turned 1.6 million American people into patients.

During the same year, The Joint National Committee on High Blood Pressure redefined hypertension requiring pharmacological intervention. Though a diastolic pressure greater than 100 mm Hg used to be considered hypertension, the value is now 90; for the systolic pressure they decreased the value from 160 to 140. This change meant that an additional 13 million Americans would require treatment.

The same pattern took place with cholesterol. Treatment used to be recommended for people with cholesterol over 300. The threshold was lowered to 240, and later fell to any measure "greater than 200." This change added 42 million people who were now target patients for the drug companies. It is important to note that the head of the diabetes panel was a paid consultant to Aventis Pharmaceuticals, Bristol-Myers Squibb, Eli Lilly, Glaxo Smith Kline, Novartis, Merck, and Pfizer—all of which make diabetes drugs.

Nine of the eleven authors of the recent blood pressure guidelines had some kind of financial ties—as paid consultants, paid speakers, or grant recipients—to drug companies that make high blood pressure drugs. Similarly, eight of nine experts who lowered the cholesterol cutoff were paid consultants to companies making cholesterol-lowering drugs.[3]

We talk about advances in health care, yet the general health of our population is not improving. According to the Word Health Organization of the United Nations, the United States of America and Canada, which have great resources of scientific minds and technology, are not at the top of the healthiest countries in the world. As health care systems go, The WHO ranks Canada as having the 30th best health care system in the world, and positions the U.S. at 37th.

Under the heading "World's Healthiest Countries," Bloomberg rankings positions the U.S. at 33rd, Canada at 14th, and Australia at 3rd.

2. Marcia Angell, MD. *The Truth About Drug Companies* (Random House, New York), 2005.
3. Dr. H. Gilbert Welch. *Over-Diagnosed: Making People Sick in the Pursuit of Health* (Beacon Press, Boston), 2011.

Dr. Albert Einstein said:

"You cannot solve cannot solve the problems of today with the same level of thinking with which they were created."

Therefore, we must encourage all politicians, taxpayers, and health care professionals to endorse the wisdom shared in this book, and move toward a health care system that embraces and respects the human body's Innate ability to heal.

"The doctor of the future will give no medicine but will interest his patients in the care of the human frame, in diet, and in the cause and prevention of disease."

THOMAS EDISON

INTRODUCTION
Dr. Gilles LaMarche

This book will challenge some of your beliefs about health and healing. You will find yourself questioning what you have learned about health from your family, friends, physicians, school teachers, and others. The health care system in North America and other developed countries is in serious trouble. In both the United States and Canada, more money per capita is spent on health care than in any other country. We have become the product of commercialized propaganda and have made many decisions about health that actually lead to *increased* disease and morbidity.

The Global Burden of Diseases' (GBD) 2010 study is a collaborative project led by the Institute for Health Metrics and Evaluation (IHME) at the University of Washington in Seattle. This major international study, published in May 2013, revealed that Australians live longer, healthier lives than people in almost every other country. Life expectancy increased for both men and women in Australia from 1990 to 2010. Australia ranks 5th out of 187 countries, with only people in Japan, Andorra, Iceland, and Switzerland living longer.

A big risk, however, is that too many people are eating, drinking, and drugging themselves to death. On average, a newborn girl in Australia can expect to live 83.8 years and a boy 79.2 years. In 1990, Australian women, on average, lived to be 80 and men died younger than 74. Men rank fifth in terms of healthy life expectancy and women rank 10th. Australians enjoy more healthy years than Americans, Britons, and New Zealanders. Australians have enjoyed significantly improved health from 1990 to 2010.

Melbourne's Professor Alan Lopez said, "We can thank two decades of campaigns by state and federal governments for driving down deaths from road injury, sudden infant death syndrome (SIDS), and tobacco."

Obesity has surpassed smoking as a risk factor. Heart disease is the leading cause of death and disability for Australians, with poor diet being the biggest risk factor. Lung cancer and stroke are next on the list, and drug abuse, depression and Alzheimer's disease are on the rise. Alzheimer's disease has increased from 26th place in 1990 to ninth in 2010 as a cause of premature death.

Dr. Christopher Murray stated, "Australia clearly has much to be proud of, however, the number of years of health loss due to obesity, alcohol, and drug use are increasing. In particular, Australians are grappling with soaring rates of obesity due to poor diet and physical inactivity."

Other concerns are high blood sugar and cholesterol.

"Policy makers and health experts must focus on the remaining threats to health," he said.[1]

To achieve better results with your health, you must be willing to think differently, look at options available, and make wiser decisions. *The ART of Being Healthy: Wellness Concepts From the Pros* is about bringing the truth to the surface and acknowledging that medicine, BIG Pharma, and the media can no longer expect to rule people with lies and deception. Many reputable and highly regarded researchers have provided information to governments that could serve to improve the health of our communities and save taxpayers billions of dollars. Few of these ideas ever get implemented. Documentaries such as *Doctored, Undoctored,* and *Making a Killing: The Untold Story of Psychotropic Drugging* present facts that are hard to believe—but fatal to ignore.

What will you do with this new information to enhance your health and that of your family?

About the Author

DR. GILLES LAMARCHE was born and raised in Timmins, Ontario, Canada. A Bachelor of Science graduate of the University of Toronto (1975), he went on to graduate with a Doctor of Chiropractic degree from Toronto's Canadian Memorial Chiropractic College in 1979. After twenty-five years of active practice, Dr. LaMarche shared his passion and talents at Parker University in Dallas, and with Parker Seminars attendees around the globe, from 2006 to 2012. In August of 2013, he accepted the position of Vice President of Professional Relations at Life University, in Atlanta, Georgia. His unequivocal passion to share health information allowing people to make informed health care choices for themselves and their families has led him to write numerous books and articles, and to share his knowledge and wisdom with audiences around the world.

The Art of Being Healthy is part of his communication strategy to allow multiple chiropractors to share their wisdom with an international audience.

For more information or to book Dr. LaMarche as a speaker at your next health and wellness event, visit his website:

www.gilleslamarche.com

1. http://www.theage.com.au/national/australians-shine-in-world-health-rankings-20130501-2iss4.html

To all the children of the world
who are born wise and pure,

To their parents who seek wisdom
in making proper choices,

To all healers who seek to
help human beings thrive,

To all teachers who persevere,

To all mentors who help raise the bar,

To all patients who give healers
enlightenment and courage to continue,

And to you, our readers, for your willing-
ness to learn and make better choices.

*"Many receive advice,
only the wise profit from it."*

Syrus

"At the heart of Chiropractic is the spinal adjustment. The chiropractor, in attempting to restore and maintain optimum health, locates and corrects spinal subluxations to enhance nervous system function. This corrective process is called a *spinal adjustment.*"

GILLES A. LAMARCHE, DC

The ART of
Being
Healthy

Our goal is to bring forth knowledge and information that will guide you to experience increased health and well-being.

CHAPTER ONE
You Were Designed Perfectly

Dr. Ryan French

Practicing in the small town of Caledon, Ontario, Canada, I have the unique privilege of serving in one of the largest Chiropractic clinics in the world. People come from hours away for our care. I believe it is because our core philosophy resonates with them.

We believe that people are designed perfectly; that health is the normal and natural state of our bodies; and that the role of a doctor is to help remove any interference to the healing process while honoring that people have the natural ability to heal from the inside.

"Every patient carries her or his own doctor inside."
ALBERT SCHWEITZER, MD, PHILOSOPHER

Don't you find it amazing that right now, without even thinking about it, your heart is beating, your lungs are breathing, your food is digesting, your liver is filtering your blood, your temperature and blood pressure are being regulated, and you are making brand-new skin cells, kidney cells, and muscle cells from the food you ate just a few hours ago? I do. In fact, after more than twenty years studying the human body, I am more amazed than ever at the intricate detail with which we are designed. Wow!

To that end, we believe that a true health care service must be directed at helping patients put their inner doctor to work so they can heal from the inside out—hence the name of our office: Inside Out Family Chiropractic.

When first introduced to this idea, most everyone agrees with it. It seems self-explanatory. It resonates with them. In fact, it seems naturally obvious. However, it is the application of this principle that most people have difficulty accomplishing.

1

Let me assure you that people who have the greatest abundance in life have figured out how to apply this principle in all areas of their lives! In this chapter, I'll discuss how to apply this from a health perspective.

I want you to be inwardly directed, to restore your belief in yourself, and give you the tools to live an amazing, abundant life, from the inside out! Your ability to be healthy is far greater than anyone has led you to believe.

Let's get started.

Can You See the Perfection?

I want you to think about a simple houseplant.

When I speak to groups around the world about health, I often ask people: *When you observe a plant that is wilting, what questions immediately come to your mind?* The answers are always the same:

"Is it getting enough water?"

"Is it getting enough sunlight?"

"Is it protected from environmental stress—abnormal temperatures or wind?"

"Is the soil healthy?"

Do those questions make sense to you? I bet they do! We all see the perfection in a plant. We know that a plant has the Innate ability to bounce back, and that healthy is its normal state. That plants are, in fact, designed to be healthy. The LIFE in the plant is always perfect if the fundamental needs of the plant are met.

If a plant has wilting leaves, we don't automatically look for some abstract diagnostic name or label that has nothing to do with the main underlying cause. We don't look at a wilting plant and try to figure out if it's "wilty leafitis" or some other name that merely just describes the symptom. No! Our thought process goes directly to the fundamental needs because of our belief that the plant already has the ability to be perfect.

We Innately know that LIFE loves LIFE.

This understanding of health can actually be applied to all living things. LIFE always strives towards health and balance. But, LIFE also has fundamental underlying requirements. If these are not met, the consequences are enormous. If these are met, LIFE flourishes.

The solution for a wilting plant is so obvious. You simply address whichever of the fundamental needs are not being met. You add water, change the soil, or alter the amount of sunlight or temperature accordingly. Simple!

Let me repeat: you address whichever of the fundamental needs are not being met.

But—and this is a huge BUT—why don't we see ourselves in the same way? Our society tends to complicate this principle when it comes to human health. Why do we ask questions like this when a person is not healthy?

"What is it?"

"What do we call it?"

"How do we get rid of it?"

Many years ago, health care stopped being about addressing fundamental needs. Instead, medicine started to address the symptoms instead of the underlying cause. They started to do "patchwork" when it came to health. This type of thinking has led us on a slippery slope.

People began to take painkillers for headaches, muscle relaxants for spasms, and anti-inflammatory pills for almost anything that hurt, etc. And people did this not just in crisis, but also to get through each day. Consumption of symptom-reducing medication has risen exponentially over the last thirty years. Let me ask you:

Do you believe that the CAUSE of a headache is a deficiency in painkiller medication?

Of course, you don't. You understand that this treatment does not address the fundamental underlying cause of headaches—it just masks it.

Do you believe the CAUSE of acid reflux is a deficiency in antacid?

Again, the answer seems so simple; yet people are satisfied with simply taking antacid to treat the symptom without ever addressing the underlying cause.

The truth is that symptoms are your body's attempt at communicating with you. They are a gift. Symptoms are absolutely not enjoyable, but they are critical. Simply taking away or masking the symptom does not make you healthier; it just makes you feel better—and that is not the same thing.

True health is a restoration of normal function, a state when the body has fewer symptoms; and ideally, no symptoms at all.

It seems there is a name for every variation in human health. There are now officially over 18,000 different diseases listed in the International Classification of Disease (ICD-10); and this number is consistently on the rise.

As you may have noticed, over the last thirty years, there is a subsequent increase in the number of medications available to treat each condition. Although some medical breakthroughs are amazing, especially as they pertain to crisis care, in general, are we getting healthier? New findings suggest that people today are being diagnosed with disease 33% faster than their grandparents. Age thirty has become the new forty-five in reference to the onset of disease. Wow.

Even though we have more health "care" available than ever before, our country is quickly sliding down the scale of the healthiest countries in the world. Neither Canada nor the U.S. rank in the top 25 countries in the world. The World Health Organization has Canada ranked 30ᵗʰ and the USA ranked 37ᵗʰ in the world for health.

To make matters worse, North Americans consume a disturbing amount of medication; the latest government statistics from Health Canada shows that Canadians fill an average of fourteen prescriptions per person per year! *Not* OK!

To put this in perspective, if my family of six fills zero prescriptions in a year, that means that another family of six is filling twenty-eight prescriptions per person to average out at fourteen per year! It seems impossible, and yet those are the statistics in Canada (the U.S. is not any better).

Realize this number does not include over-the-counter medications, just prescription meds. Canadian seniors, sixty-five to eighty years of age, average a new prescription every ten days, and Canadians over eighty average a new prescription every three to four days! Wow!

"If all the medicine in the world were thrown into the sea, it would be bad for the fish and good for humanity."
OLIVER WENDELL HOLMES, MD

Don't get me wrong; there is a time and place for crisis management. In fact, I think it is an amazing gift that so many people have been helped in crisis by medication. Drugs and surgery are second to none in crisis management.

But I want to be clear: that which is good for you in crisis does not help you create long-term health. At some point, it became "normal" for people to carry pills in their purses and in their cars. At some point, it became OK for pharmaceutical companies to advertise drugs directly to people and encourage them to ask their doctors in the hope that they would sell more product.

I wonder, have you ever known someone who was admitted

into a nursing home, given all that medication, gotten better, and returned home? I doubt it.

The truth is that treating symptoms rarely, if ever, produces true health. We are truly on a slippery slope when it comes to health care. Our health care system is failing miserably because it doesn't address underlying causes. It is broken—and humanity deserves better. It starts with remembering how amazing the human body is.

We all need to understand that our day-to-day decisions are based on our personal belief systems. If you believe that the human body is inherently weak, that it has little or no ability to heal itself, then it makes perfect sense that you would turn to something from the outside in, in order to help you get past a symptom.

If you believe that the human body is inherently strong, that it has great ability to heal itself, then it makes perfect sense that you would turn to something that helps your body heal naturally, which, in turn, leads to normal resolution of the symptom.

Children who grow up believing they are weak, will learn the habit of looking to the outside for answers; in all areas, not just health.

Children who grow up believing they are inherently and naturally strong, will learn the habit of looking inward for answers; in all areas. This is what I want for my kids. How about you?

You Are Amazing

My wife and I have been blessed with four beautiful children. Watching them being born, taking their first breath, finding the breast without instruction, and watching them grow has brought me to tears on more than one occasion. I am so grateful.

The miracle of LIFE is beautiful. In fact, most people agree on this, especially when looking at a baby. Most look at babies in AWE. In fact, we usually say awwww when we look at baby pictures or see a little one. Don't we?

I need your attention here. You need to remember that YOU are still a miracle of LIFE. You came from two cells, one from your mom and one from your dad. About nine months later, you were seventy trillion cells, nine organ systems, and seven pounds and twenty-two inches or so of pure miracle. Amazing!

You did not stop being a miracle just because you grew up. No! You are still amazing.

At the beginning, just after conception, the first things to form are the central axis, the brain and spinal cord. The brain and spinal cord are first as they become the central command center for development and function. This happens before the woman even knows she is pregnant!

Within weeks, the heart is formed, and the gut tract is too. One by one, the organs develop, all connected to the central command center via the developing nerves. Everyone looks at the details of development with amazement. When it comes to newborns, we are in a state of awe and wonder.

And here's what most people forget: this same intelligence that knitted you together does not leave when you enter the world. This organizing intelligence remains as Innate Intelligence, the intelligence responsible for the coordination of LIFE within you.

> "That power which set the Universe in motion and created me did not abandon me when I became free of the security of my earthly mother's womb. It is still with me and protects me as it moves all forms toward their final predestined goal. It is not mine to educatedly ask 'why' or 'where', but to Innately live; and live to help my fellow creatures."
>
> DR. B. J. PALMER

Right now, this Innate Intelligence is controlling and coordinating everything! Your heart will beat around 100,000 times today. You will breathe fifteen breaths per minute. Your body temperature will stay around thirty-seven degrees Celsius, and your blood pH level will maintain at 7.4. You will make 200 billion new red blood cells and 400 billion new platelets today. You will make brand-new kidney cells, heart cells, stomach cells, and toenails from the food you ate yesterday! Amazing!

> "The function of Innate Intelligence is to adapt universal forces and matter for use in the body, so that all parts of the body will have co-ordinate action for mutual benefit."
>
> R. W. STEPHENSON, 1927

There is an internal intelligence that guides this perfect process. People have different ideas about what to call this intelligence, and even different ideas about where it came from. I believe that God breathes that LIFE into us. Some call it *Mother Nature*. The Chinese call this power *Chi*, and Indian culture calls it *Prana*. I have heard it called the *life force* or the *vital force*, and chiropractors call it *Innate Intelligence*. For the purposes of simplicity, I'll just call it *LIFE*. Regardless of what you call it, we need to recognize that there is an intelligence that runs our bodies and whose power exceeds our understanding.

Thank goodness you don't have to remember to breathe, to make new cells, to digest your food. Thank goodness LIFE happens on its own! You need to trust this.

Fundamental Needs

In the earlier example, you knew that a wilting plant must be missing one of its fundamental needs.

Likewise, the human body has four fundamental requirements for survival. These are: water, air, food, and LIFE. Without any one of these, the human body cannot survive.

Humans can live several weeks without food, days without water, minutes without air, and just milliseconds without LIFE. In medical analysis, LIFE is measured by brainwave activity.

They even have names for them, three of which I am sure you are familiar with, and one that I need to introduce you to:

A lack of water is called *dehydration*.

A lack of air is called *suffocation*.

A lack of nutrition is called *malnutrition*.

A lack of LIFE is called *subluxation*.

Subluxation is a Chiropractic term that means an interference to the normal flow of LIFE in the body.

"**Sub**" means less than or under
"**Lux**" means light or life
"**Ation**" means condition
So, SUBLUXATION means:

**A condition of less than full light;
or a condition of less than full LIFE.**

When I examine a patient, I want to know one simple thing: is there any way I can help this person's body work closer to the way it was designed? I look for any subluxation in the spine and nerve system. I am not trying to only find out how to make him or her just feel better; I need to get him to HEAL better.

I look at the requirements of the body and determine which of the fundamental needs are not being met. As a health educator, I often address the first three: plenty of water, plenty of exercise, and proper nutrition. Of course, anyone making a change in one of these three areas will have some health benefit. Most often, people can do this on their own.

As a practicing chiropractor, my sole function is to address sub-luxation. If I can find a subluxation and remove it, the body will automatically resume control and LIFE will start to heal the body on its own.

Anatomy 101

You have an amazing brain that comes with its own built-in helmet: the skull. Why do you suppose God protects the entire brain with bone? Because this is where LIFE flows from. If your brain dies, the rest of you will die. There isn't anything within the realm of the human experience that doesn't involve the brain.

LIFE flows from the brain to the body, and vice versa, through the spinal cord and thirty-three pairs of nerves. This system operates like the Internet, where the brain sends messages through the nerves to all the different parts of the body.

Like the brain, the spinal cord is critically important, which is why you were designed with a series of special bones stacked on top of one another with a continuous hole down the middle where the spinal cord sits. These spinal bones, called *vertebrae*, are there to protect that very delicate spinal cord.

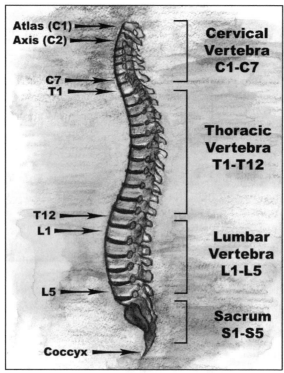

Figure 1. The human spine.

There are four general regions of the spine: the cervical (neck), thoracic (mid-back), lumbar (low back) and sacral (pelvis) regions. Knowing exactly where the nerves go, will help you understand your health and your body much better.

Cervical Spine (C1 to C7)

The nerves from the neck supply LIFE to the head and neck, eyes, ears, nose, throat, sinuses, neck muscles, thyroid, and into the shoulders, arms, and hands. If someone has a subluxation in the neck, it can lead to problems as indicated in the following chart. Look for health problems that you might have; or that someone in your family might have.

Region	Areas and Parts of the Body	Possible Symptoms
Neck	Nerves from the neck region go around the head, eyes, ears, nose, throat, thyroid, neck muscles, shoulders, down the arms, and into the hands	Subluxations in the neck can lead to headaches, migraines, insomnia, chronic ear and sinus infections, ringing in the ears, swollen tonsils and adenoids, thyroid conditions, numbness in hands, and more

For someone with a subluxation in the neck, the most common symptoms are headaches, neck pain, or tingling in the fingers. In an outside-in clinic, which is philosophically opposite to our inside-out clinic, the patient would typically receive a painkiller for the headache, a muscle relaxant for the muscle pain, and an anti-inflammatory for the numbness. Of course, none of these remedies ever gets to the actual underlying cause of the symptom.

Thoracic Spine (T1-T12)

The nerves in the mid-back supply LIFE to the area between the shoulder blades, the shoulders, the chest wall, the lungs, the heart, and the upper part of the stomach. If someone has a subluxation in the mid-back, it can lead to health problems as indicated in the following chart. Do you know anyone who has any of these?

Region	Areas and Parts of the Body	Possible Symptoms
Mid-Back	Nerves from the mid-back go around the mid-section, between the shoulder blades, the ribs, heart, lungs, and the upper part of the stomach	Subluxations in the mid-back can lead to tightness between the shoulder blades, chronic shoulder pain, heart problems, chronic chest infection, asthma acid reflux, and more

Lumbar Spine and Pelvis (L1-L5 and Sacrum)

The nerves in the low back supply LIFE to the lower back, down the legs, and all the organs in the lower abdomen and pelvic area. Anyone who has had low-back pain knows that in some cases it can radiate down the leg in a very painful condition known as sciatica. Ouch! This is one of the most painful conditions.

Region	Areas and Parts of the Body	Possible Symptoms
Low-Back	Nerves from the lower back go around the hips, down the buttock, into the legs, lower digestive organs, sex organs, bladder, feet, and muscles of the lower back	Subluxations in the mid-back can lead to sciatica, pain in the hips, numbness in the legs to the feet and toes, constipation, bowel gas, bloating, menstrual cramping, sex organ dysfunction, and more

If you or anyone you know suffers from any of these health conditions, the underlying cause may be subluxation in the nerve system. A highly trained doctor of Chiropractic will be able to determine this.

The Flow of LIFE

In a normal circumstance, LIFE flows between the brain and body via the spinal cord and nerves, at all times. Normal communication results in the creation of health.

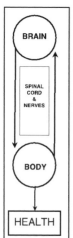

The graphic at the left indicates the critical connection between the brain and the body for the production of health. If there is interference to this connection, your body begins a predictable breakdown pattern. This interference is caused by subluxation.

The first thing that happens is that the body shifts from a state of EASE to a state of DIS-EASE.

DIS-EASE is a lack of LIFE, lack of balance, a lack of harmony, a lack of adaptability, and a lack of normalcy.

Some people in a state of DIS-EASE will experience symptoms. Notice that I said *some*, not all—which is why this process needs to be closely evaluated. You simply cannot rely on how you feel as an indicator of your health.

Have you ever heard of someone having a heart attack with no prior symptoms?

Have you ever heard of someone diagnosed with cancer on a routine screening?

Have you ever heard of someone diagnosed with high blood pressure or high cholesterol even though they feel fine?

Of course, you have. The point is simple: your body doesn't always exhibit a symptom; and sometimes, when you notice a symptom it is too late. The other point is: The only way to know if you are subluxated is to be examined by someone who is trained to detect and correct subluxations. Right now, the only professionals trained to do this are chiropractors. A medical doctor has minimal hours training in anatomy and neurology compared to a chiropractor who specializes in this. Medical doctors simply specialize in something different.

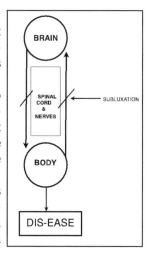

A complete examination for subluxation involves a thorough history, Chiropractic physical examination, computerized stress testing, and often x-ray evaluation. (For more details about a typical first examination with a chiropractor, visit www.insideoutchiro.org and click on the New Patient section.)

The Transition from DIS-EASE to DISEASE

If you have pressure on the nerves disturbing the flow of LIFE for an extended period of time, your body will make the transition from DIS-EASE to full on DISEASE. Here is a simple illustration. Grab and squeeze your left index finger with your right hand, leaving the tip of your index finger exposed. Notice that there is an instant change in the color of the tip of your finger. Can you imagine that after five minutes this might begin to feel uncomfortable? The tip of your finger will turn dark red, maybe even purple, in that time period. Welcome to the state of DIS-EASE. The finger isn't working perfectly, but it's definitely still bearable and is not damaged long-term.

Imagine if you held it for three months. There would be more damage. The fingernail would turn dark purple, then black, and eventually fall off. It would become more susceptible to disease, and the symptoms of this process would likely increase.

Welcome to the state of DISEASE. The only difference between a lack of EASE and complete DISEASE is TIME! It's actually the same problem, but has become chronic.

Chiropractors want to free people from ever experiencing the effects of chronic subluxation.

Since many people don't take care of themselves until something hurts, many show up in our office in health crisis thinking that the problem just began. Not true! They bend over to pick up a shoe and their lower back goes out. They believe that one event caused the damage.

You must understand that the simple process of bending over is not enough to break down a grown man's back—but rather it is the proverbial straw that broke the camel's back. It was that one extra stress that the body simply couldn't handle, because it was ALREADY in a state of DIS-EASE for a period of time.

For you to get and stay healthy, it is critical to deal with body imbalances BEFORE they enter the disease state.

The Adjustment

A specific Chiropractic *adjustment* is designed to remove any subluxation in the spine; to remove all interference to the flow of LIFE. Regular Chiropractic adjustments will keep you free of interference throughout your lifetime.

This is what we offer in our office.

"ad" means addition or moving toward an indicated direction
"just" means made according to principle or guided by truth
"ment" means indicating an action or resulting state
So ADJUSTMENT means:

**Moving towards a state of being
guided by truth, according to principle.**

The first principle in Chiropractic, known as the *Major Premise*, states:

"A Universal Intelligence is in all matter and continually
gives to it all its properties and actions,
thus maintaining it in existence."
DR. R. W. STEPHENSON

An adjustment moves you towards a state of being guided by Innate Intelligence. It allows your body to function, heal, and re-create on a continual basis with amazing perfection.

In my office, I have one goal for all patients: to move them towards living free of chronic subluxation.

Chiropractic adjustments can be applied to anyone with a spine: newborns, children, adolescents, adults, and seniors alike. In our office, we have a special interest in taking care of families, and have extensive education with respect to pediatrics, growth, and development.

We know:

It is way easier to raise a healthy child than it is to repair a damaged adult!

Chiropractic adjustments can be done using our hands, with special tables, specific adjusting instruments, and more. We always find a way that is comfortable and effective for every person we meet. Since no two people are alike, the application of the adjustment is different depending on each case.

"Your health and life is coordinated and expressed through your nerve system. A Chiropractic adjustment removes interference to the perfect programming you already have. It has nothing to do with a bummed knee or heart disease except that these are signs of your perfect expression going wrong."

Dr. Matthew Tonnos

Termites?

Why are termites dangerous in a home? Simple: they can eat away at the foundation and cause significant damage BEFORE you ever discover they are there. You may see one or two hanging around, but you might not understand or recognize that those few termites you see are NOT the problem—it's the thousands of others that are hidden that cause all the damage!

This is like a subluxation in the spine. Recall that a subluxation is a misalignment in the spine that interferes with the nerves and flow of LIFE, and causes premature breakdown and decay on the inside. *Not* OK.

Like termites, the damage of subluxations is almost always significant BEFORE you ever discover they are there. Subluxations cause the body to begin a predictable breakdown process. If subluxations are detected early enough, like termites, they can very simply be corrected to avoid serious damage. This is what a Chiropractic adjustment does.

One of the greatest benefits to regular Chiropractic care is the countless number of health challenges that it helps prevent. Yes, Chiropractic care can help once there is damage, but it's true value takes place long before damage/symptoms occur.

For example, recently I examined an asymptomatic man with 83% loss of normal alignment on the inside. Even though he was developing multiple degenerating discs and bone spurs, he didn't know about it—just like having termites in your foundation. The amazing value for this man will be the correction of this underlying problem before it ever turns into severe disability and disease. Awesome!

Subluxation alone is enough reason to find a chiropractor and utilize his/her services for you and your family, for a lifetime. You will be glad you did!

Always remember: you are amazing. You are designed with perfection. You are designed to enjoy health in abundance. You are designed to enjoy LIFE!

I encourage you to seek out a chiropractor in your area who is dedicated to helping families be amazing. If you have trouble finding one, email me directly at DrRyan@insideoutchiro.org, I am happy to help you find someone great!

Please visit our website www.insideoutchiro.org for more information or call us directly at 905-951-9911.

About the Author

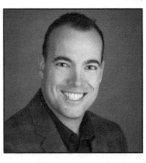

DR. RYAN FRENCH is a family chiropractor practicing in Bolton, Ontario. Together with his amazing team of support staff and associate doctors, he has built the largest family wellness center in the area. He is a health coach, teacher, and writer.

Dr. Ryan received his doctorate from the Canadian Memorial Chiropractic College in Toronto. His other academic accomplishments include a Degree in Kinesiology (the science of the Human Body) from McMaster University in Hamilton; a post-doctorate fellowship in pregnancy and pediatric care providing him the title FICPA (Fellow of the International Chiropractic Pediatric Association); certification in The Webster In-Utero Constraint Technique (better known as the breech-turning technique); certification to practice Clinical Acupuncture; and many other courses in nutrition, exercise, and preventive health care.

He is blessed with a wonderful family, including his loving wife, Suzanne, and four beautiful children, Jessica, Jackson, Jordyn, and Jacob. His hobbies include coaching, hockey, fishing, golf, and never-ending learning!

You can also contact Dr. French at:

Inside Out Family Chiropractic
27 King Street East
Bolton, Ontario
Phone: (905) 951-9911
Email: drryan@insideoutchiro.org

CHAPTER TWO
The Evolution of Your Revolution

Dr. Robert Kipp

Do you ever think about the journey required to get anywhere in life? I think about the challenges, successes, and changes that have occurred in my life. I think about how they impacted not only me, but the lives of others whom I've come in contact with. How, if I had made different decisions, things would be different right this very instant. Oftentimes, people look back on decisions with regret, but this is not what I am referring to. I am referring to lessons that you can learn from and utilize to improve your life.

One of the beauties of our evolution as human beings is the power of choice. How does the power of choice relate to being healthy?

Each day, you are presented with hundreds, if not thousands, of different choices. These seemingly harmless choices all add together to dictate your current health status. Think about what you ate for breakfast, what shoes you decided to wear, how long you will sit during the day, whether you choose to exercise or not, and whether you are optimistic or in a slump. These are just a few of the choices you are given every day. Each decision you make may seem insignificant by itself, but the cumulative effect on your overall health can be enormous—especially if you continuously make poor choices day after day.

Your ability to think about, and direct, your own wellness revolution lies within these daily choices. Everyone experiences challenges, successes, failures, and changes during their quest for better health, but as long as the successes outnumber the failures, the positive evolution of your revolution is taking place.

Before we get into the nuts and bolts of shifting your health consciousness, I want to be completely honest with you. I haven't always made the healthiest lifestyle choices. I've made some poor health choices because I didn't know any better, but also because I perceived that the pain of changing my routine was harder to handle than the reward of the change itself. Some poor choices took place during my younger rebellious phase, but there were also times when I knew what the better choice was and either stayed stuck in my rut or disregarded the obvious.

In other words, chances are I've probably been where you are now. Don't get me wrong, I am truly grateful for the experiences that have brought me to this place of good health and well-being. It is because I have experienced the effects of both bad and good choices that I can now offer some perspective on how to evaluate your decision-making process. I am hopeful you will take some of these concepts and use them to positively affect your life and that of your family.

Let me first take you back a number of years. To say I was a bit of a challenge as a kid would be the understatement of the century! If there was a dare, I'd take it; something dangerous, count me in; an obstacle, I'd make it through. For the most part, these headstrong tendencies would help me tremendously when I came to realize that I could use them as strengths—but this evolution would not come quickly or easily.

If you can think of ways to abuse your body, I probably tried them at some point in my journey. As I look back on these pivotal educational moments, there are a few that stand out from the rest, ones I would consider game-changers. These are the points that can propel a change in your life that will take you to a much healthier place if you decide you are ready. A few of my game-changing moments included the day I fell out of a tree, the moment I quit smoking cigarettes, and the time I was able to make valuable reflections during my grandmother's illness. I know these seem like major events, and they were. I hope you'll come to realize that life events are presented in order for people to learn and grow.

There is a catch though. You can decide to make a change or you can decide to do nothing and stay the same. The choice is always up to you. It was Albert Einstein who said, "Doing the same thing the same way and expecting different results is a sign of insanity."

One rainy Friday afternoon, in the fall of 1994, a game-changing moment occurred that created a transformative shift in my life. I had finished my classes in the early afternoon and decided to take a trip to my friend's house in upstate New York. I had always loved fishing and hunting, and this was the time of year to get ready for deer hunting season. So, out to the woods I went to set up my tree stand. Everything was going as planned, until I slipped. Unable to catch myself, I fell about fifteen feet and landed on a rock. I knew I was hurt, but I had no idea of the extent.

Looking back, I remember thinking, "I'm going to wait and see if I really need to go to the hospital." I am not advocating for this type of thinking, because I realize now it was really stupid! After a few days of sheer agony, I ended up in the emergency room with a broken shoulder blade, collar bone, and several broken ribs. As a know-it-all premed student, my discussion with the attending orthopedic surgeon was quite comical. I began throwing around words like *diagnosis* and *prognosis*. (I am sure he wasn't amused.) While we talked, my eyes were opened to something profound: if I had all the recommended surgeries, or if I opted for NO surgeries, my prognosis (outcome) was almost identical! How could this be? I wondered. The answer was the game-changer. Logically, I chose the route with no surgery involved. But I knew that I still needed help; so I called my mom for some guidance. She recommended that I go to her chiropractor. I took her advice and scheduled an appointment.

At my first appointment, I was handed a series of forms to complete and then told to have a seat. Not long after, I was escorted to an examination room and told that the doctor would be right in. To my surprise, a woman standing about four feet five inches tall came in and introduced herself as my chiropractor. After discussing my dilemma, and going through a thorough examination, this short, female said in a thick accent, "If you give your body what it needs, it will take care of you." Simple, yet perfect.

I didn't realize it at the time, but her statement would become the foundation for all of the care programs I would put together for my future patients.

She proceeded to walk me through the steps that my body required for healing—and today, I am happy to say, that the only remnant of that terrible accident is a right shoulder that is one inch lower than my left. No aches, no pains, no loss of function. I followed her recommendations and gave my body what it needed. Thank God for my Chiropractor!

This experience began to shift my career views almost immediately, but I continued on with my premed studies nonetheless. About a year later, while still in school, I met my future wife, Susan. She and I often spoke about my possible career as an orthopedic surgeon, and then something happened. Susan challenged me the way people who love us frequently do. She questioned my decision to focus on orthopedic surgery when, in fact, it was Chiropractic that had changed my life. These late-night conversations came to a head when she finally came out and asked, "Why don't you become a chiropractor?"

At this time, I had thought of it a bit, but nothing more. We discussed this possibility further and Susan brought up so many points that metaphorically hit me right over the head: I am supposed to be a chiropractor!

Thus, I went to Chiropractic college, married my college sweetheart, and now have a wonderful practice in which we are able to help people understand the biggest fundamental truth in health: THE BODY HAS THE INNATE ABILITY TO HEAL ITSELF! This will always be true as long as you give your body what it needs and, at the same time, keep the interference to a minimum.

I will share some examples of what your body needs later, but right now, let's take a look at another game-changing concept that stops so many people from being healthier: habits.

I am going to share something that I am not proud of, especially as a preacher of health. When I was about fifteen years old, one of my good friends showed up at our after-school meeting spot with a pack of cigarettes. Now, I happen to have a very outgoing personality that has a great deal of positive attributes, but it also contains pitfalls that I need to watch out for. In this case, the pitfall was that I didn't want to be the one who didn't try something.

So began my habit of smoking. As a teenager, I never gave much thought to the long-term effects that smoking would have on my health. I was much more concerned with the here and now and the things that would give me pleasure. The feeling I got from the nicotine certainly hit that pleasure center. Over the next several years, a very noticeable pattern emerged. I would smoke after eating and while I was out with my friends. I would smoke when I felt stressed or when I was taking a ride in the car. Despite all the warnings on the box and the television commercials, I kept doing what I had trained myself to do. (I am embarrassed to admit that I kept up this habit even after becoming a Doctor of Chiropractic; despite knowing the truth.)

I heard so many horror stories of people who tried to quit and failed, that I figured why bother? I won't smoke as much. I won't smoke during my patient hours. This is the way I rationalized continuing to do what I knew was bad for me.

Do you see the problem here? I had developed unhealthy habits that I was unwilling to change, and at the same time I was telling people how to be healthy. WHY?

It took me years to understand this second fundamental truth: "If we perceive the pain of changing to be greater than the pleasure of the action, we will not make a change." The thought of changing all of my daily routines that I had built around smoking cigarettes was far more painful than the joy I perceived I would gain by quitting.

All of us do this, whether we realize it or not. We have an amazing ability to convince ourselves that our choices are the right ones.

We also have the ability to make excuses if they are not. This is why people like you and me sometimes get stuck in a rut when it comes to making changes in our lives.

Fast forward to an afternoon in Cincinnati, Ohio, where I was attending a Chiropractic conference. I was seated about fifteen rows back in the center of the crowd. I had decided to attend this conference on a last-minute decision, but it would prove to be one of the most valuable decisions I've ever made (maybe like your decision to read this book!). I was in a lecture being given by my colleague Dr. Patrick Gentempo. It was during this hour and a half that he had us do an exercise that changed my life forever. He said, and I paraphrase, "I want you to close your eyes and think about something that you'd like to change in your life. Now, picture how your life would be different. How would you be different? How would your relationships change? Think about all the good things that would come from making that change. Now that you have that image, all that is standing in your way of having that life, is you doing it."

My desire was to stop smoking. It would improve my life in all areas—I just had to do it. After the session, I walked outside and threw away what was left in my pack of cigarettes and have never looked back. There were certainly difficult times afterward, but my desire to create the image I saw in my mind that day overpowered my desire to start again. Charles Duhigg, author of the book *The Power of Habit* puts it perfectly. He says: "Willpower isn't just a skill. It's like a muscle in your arms or legs, and it gets tired as it works harder, so there's less power left over for other things."

When you decide to make changes in your lifestyle in order to be healthier, you must understand that some things will be difficult. However, if you keep doing the exercise that Dr. Gentempo had the audience do, you will stay connected to your higher values and it will give you the strength to keep pushing forward.

You have the power to change any habit that you currently have, as long as you value the outcome.

When you first decide to make changes, it helps to write down the new choices you are making and to let others know. These two things will support your choices and hold you accountable for them. Don't worry if you slip up. If this happens, acknowledge it and figure out why it happened. This will help you overcome the same obstacle that is sure to show up again and again. And, be willing to ask for help when you need it. Your support system is crucial to your success, and the people in your circle of influence are there to help you achieve the results you want.

And, here's the second game-changing thought: YOU HAVE THE CHOICE TO BE HEALTHIER BY CHOOSING TO DO HEALTHIER

THINGS. YOU HAVE THE CHOICE TO BE HEALTHIER BY MAKING BETTER HEALTH CHOICES. Let's move on to the third game-changer. Several years ago, my wife and I received a call that no one ever wants to get. My younger sister, a nurse at Albany Medical Center in New York, called to let us know that our grandmother was taken to the hospital because her behavior had changed drastically that day and my grandfather didn't know what to do. After a series of tests and scans, a brain tumor was discovered. Our grandparents have always been a big part of our lives; so this news was shocking and devastating.

The reason I bring this up is not to focus on the fact that my grandmother had taken ill, but to illustrate a point that became obvious to me at that time. When a major life event takes place, the trivial day-to-day things become minimized and we can clearly see the things that actually matter. As my family continued to go through this journey with Gram, it became evident that there was something that was constant, every minute of every day: love.

I could see it in my grandfather, my parents, my siblings, and all of my other relatives. There was love for my grandmother. Not just because she was in a hospital bed, but because of who she was and how she had touched everyone. I also realized that there was love for one another in the family as well. This love was always present—but the clarity in the absence of the trivial things was amazing. I experienced what really mattered.

The symbol of love has long been a heart. I don't believe this is random. The heart works as a pump in order to maintain life. If we simply look at the parallel, love is also required to maintain life. It has the power to change people. It has the power to make us do things that make our lives better. Love is an essential ingredient in the recipe of life. Surround yourself with people you love and with people who love you in order to have your best chances of success. When you have the support of people whom you love, and that love you, choosing to live a healthier life becomes easy.

These three game-changing moments, and their resulting concepts, have helped me lay a strong foundation for trying to master the art of being healthy.

Living healthier can be a constant battle because of the stresses of our every day of our lives. But knowing that the body has the ability to heal itself, if you give it what it needs, and knowing that you can live healthier by choosing to make healthier choices becomes more important and valuable when you consider how it impacts the ones you love. This foundation is strong and it is yours to use; however, the information that you've received thus far is only as good as the actions you take to make them your new reality.

Since 2001, when I became a chiropractor, I have been asked many times how to restore and maintain health. Eventually, I started to realize that so many of the questions emphasized the restore side of the equation. Think about this for a minute. If people first made healthy choices and then *continued to make* wise health choices, why wouldn't they keep experiencing health? If it's true that willpower is a muscle, some exercises for this muscle will go a long way in helping change some of the harder things later.

We know the body breaks down over time. But are we doing things to speed that up or slow it down? It's likely that no one has ever told you how to make the good choices and keep building on them. You see, there is no magic bullet to make you healthy. Health is a process that looks something like this: see the need for change, evaluate the choices, take action, and then evaluate the outcome. Hopefully that outcome allows you to enjoy every minute of the rest of your life with quality.

Here's the Golden Rule: Being healthy doesn't have to be difficult. If you divide your lifestyle into a few major categories and evaluate how you are doing in each, it can be a great starting point to making changes toward better health.

Let's look at the categories of mental health, nutritional health, and physical health. Most of your day-to-day choices can be placed in one of these major categories. Your choices will then go through an internal rating system in order to assign a level of personal difficulty. In other words, how hard is this choice going to be for me? This is important to realize, because the bigger the difficulty the more likely it is you will have to pay attention to it. These are things you might see as being impossible right now—like quitting smoking, starting an exercise program, or giving up alcohol. But don't worry, you can do it! We are going to start with easier changes to fuel your success; then graduate to the bigger ones.

Let's use mental health as our first category of evolution. Henry Ford said, "Whether you think you can, or think you can't, you're usually right." Right now, take a moment to close your eyes and envision what would change in your life if you were perfectly healthy. Would you be able to have more fun, play with your children more, live without pain, be more active, accomplish what you want? Now choose. Continue to live your life at your current health level or do what it takes to make it better. Your health success depends on the six inches between your ears and how you choose to use it.

Gratitude, present-time consciousness, and *forgiveness* are three concepts that can launch you in a healthy direction when used daily. Of course, there are plenty of others, but these give you a great place to start with some easy decisions.

Choose to be grateful. One of my mentors, Dr. Troy Dukowitz, taught me a technique that helps me take note of all the people in my life for whom I am grateful. He calls this a "Gratitude List." It is a simple, but profound, five-minute exercise that you can do every morning. First, take a sheet of paper and title it "Gratitude List" so that your brain knows what you are writing about. For the next five minutes, write down the names of everyone you come in contact with and for whom you are grateful. The list can include family, friends, neighbors, teachers, church members, coworkers, and staff members. There is one rule for this exercise: if you stop writing for more than three seconds, the exercise is DONE and you can do it again tomorrow. In just a few days, you will realize that your list has grown because you are more aware of gratitude. Think about how different your day can be if you did this every morning instead of watching the news!

Choose to be "in the moment." Present-time consciousness can be challenging because of the distractions all around us. Smart phones, text messaging, and tablet computers allow us to be connected to thousands of people at any moment—but what about the person standing right in front of you? Are you being present with them? Is a text message or email more important than your spouse or significant other? What about your child? Technology can be a wonderful asset, but can also make being present challenging.

Choose to be present by turning off your cell phone when you are with other people. Start easy by doing it during meals, but then expand it to include meetings, family activities, date night, and work. Imagine how connected you could get with people without that distraction.

Now, let's discuss forgiveness. For some people, forgiveness comes easily, and learning from them is the best way to make it easier for the rest of us. All of the people I have encountered who can forgive easily seem to share a common trait: they seem to view the collective good of the person and allow that to outweigh the wrong that they have done. It's not uncommon to immediately bring up the elephant in the room when working on forgiveness, but resist that temptation.

Start with smaller things to forgive and build up to the big ones. Imagine your life if you didn't hold any grudges or harbor any resentment. If that thought didn't just bring a smile to your face, think harder, because life without those negative energies is way easier and a whole lot more fun.

Now that you've eliminated some negative baggage and are thinking healthier thoughts, it's time to talk about the fuel that you power your body with. That's right, food. There are three straightforward challenges that I have for you when it comes to food: how you shop, what you eat, and how you support your food. The first challenge is fairly easy. I call it *perimeter shopping*, and it happens like this: When you go to the grocery store, make a decision to purchase things from the perimeter of the store only. Think about it. What's there? It is where the fresh fruits and vegetables, meats, and other perishable items are kept. The rule is: if something can rot in a few days if you leave it out, it's probably good for you. When you shop like this, it takes away the desire to pick up the cookies, crackers, sodas, and other things that are addictive and have a shelf life of years, not days. When in doubt, ask yourself "Is this really healthy for me?" If you have to think about it, put it back.

Next, is what you eat. This always causes controversy because people are passionate about what they believe to be right. Let me make it easy. We can use history to our advantage and think about what our ancestors ate over the last 200,000 years. If our genetic code has been formed since the beginning of time, why wouldn't we eat the same way? Here's an interesting experiment: For one month, eat the way our ancestors did. The list is short: fruits, vegetables, nuts, seeds, meat/fish, and water. If you notice, there are no dairy, grains, or artificial sugars on the list. (Also, you can find all of these foods around the perimeter of the grocery store!)

I want to address dairy because I get a lot of questions on that subject. The commercialization of milk and dairy took place over the last hundred years or so. In that time, look at how many people have developed dairy sensitivities. Just because someone is able to tolerate milk from another mammal, does not necessarily mean that it is good for you. If it's calcium you're worried about, eat more green leafy vegetables, like spinach and kale—they contain a lot of calcium. Humans are the only mammals that have chosen to consume milk from a different species. Did you ever consider this fact? Would it make sense to avoid milk products? With my experience, I must say a very loud yes.

It is also important to consider the subject of nutritional supplementation. In 2001, the American Medical Association supported a statement about the need for everyone to take a multivitamin with trace minerals because our soil has been so drastically depleted. More recently, research presented by Dr. James Chestnut, Scientist and Chiropractor, has shown the need to add vitamin D, omega-3 fatty acids from fish oil, and probiotics to help normalize the bacteria in the gut. You should consult your chiropractor to determine the brand and amount that will be best for you. Please make sure that you are supplementing.

Finally, the last major category that we need to assess is your physical health. As a chiropractor, it is the one I can directly help with the most. As I said, we started easy and left the bigger challenges for last.

The first physical action that you can take to be healthier is to simply move. Moderate exercise three to five days per week for thirty minutes each day can drastically improve EVERY SINGLE ASPECT of your body's vitality. The only decision you have to make is how you are going to move. It doesn't matter if you like to run, power walk, swim, dance, cycle, or lift weights. It just matters that you take action and do it. Scheduling time on your calendar will make this more of a reality for you and allow you to succeed. Remember to start off slowly and build. Physical improvements, along with everything else we've discussed, take time and should not be rushed.

Now, allow me to join all the pieces of the puzzle together for you with the second point. There is a system of the body that is directly involved with everything that we have talked about up. Can you name it? It is involved in thinking and feeling. It directs the stomach and intestines to break down and digest the foods you eat. It controls the muscles that you use to move and exercise. Got it yet? That's right, the nervous system!

The forty-five miles of nerves that run through your body control and coordinate every single action and process that your body does. Remember how your body has the ability to heal itself? How do you think that happens?

People can survive without food for about twenty-one days, without water up to about ten days, without air for three to five minutes—but if you cut the nerve that controls the heart, you will die instantly. The importance of the nervous system is unrivaled; and therefore, so is the maintenance of this precious system. As chiropractors, this is how we help people live healthier lives. All of the stresses that your body encounters on a daily basis are sure to cause some interference in the function of the nervous system. The body's response to these different types of stress can be seen in what is called a *vertebral subluxation*. This happens when the bones of the spine that surround the central nervous system lose their normal position or function. For every subluxation you have, your nervous system functions worse. Some people might experience things like allergies or indigestion, heart palpitations or asthma, and a variety of other signs and symptoms. If left uncorrected long enough, your body might even sound the alarm system which you experience as pain.

A chiropractor's responsibility is to find and correct these subluxations to allow your nervous system to do its job. Remember, if your body is able to heal provided you give it what it needs, what could be more important than taking care of the nervous system that gives you life from one second to the next? If you answered nothing, then you'd be correct.

The art of being healthy contains a number of moving parts and is a never-ending evolution. You are constantly challenged with stressors, and if you choose to ignore them, they will surely take your health from you. However, if you choose to recognize the stressors, make the necessary healthy decisions, and take action, you stand a much better chance of living a life filled with quality days.

Imagine what your life would look like if you did just some of the things you just read about. Can you imagine your life filled with love, health, and success?

Ask yourself this question: "When will I start the evolution of my health revolution?" Hopefully, with the information gained by reading this book, your answer is NOW.

About the Author

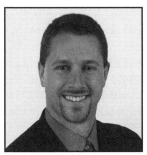

DR. ROBERT KIPP, a 2001 graduate of Northwestern College of Chiropractic, currently practices in Southport, Connecticut. He and his wife, Susan, started Pro-Health Chiropractic to help people make healthy changes in their lifestyle so they could experience a higher quality of life.

Dr. Kipp has served six years as President of the Parker GTO Club, a group of chiropractors committed to improving the profession through education and mentoring. He has been a speaker on many occasions for Chiropractic organizations as well as public and civic organizations.

Enduring the personal challenges of life has given Dr. Kipp unique perspectives on how to serve others. With the help of his wife, Dr. Kipp has assisted thousands of individuals and families achieve better health through living a Chiropractic wellness program. His passion for sharing and improving lives has most recently compelled him to co-author this book.

Dr. Kipp is available to speak on a variety of health topics for your business or club. Information about the program and practice can be found on his website: www.yourprohealth.com.

You can also contact Dr. Kipp at:

Pro-Health Chiropractic
2600 Post Road, Suite L2
Southport, CT 06890
Phone: (203) 333-2700
Email: drk@yourprohealth.com

CHAPTER THREE
How Can Chiropractic Help Me?

Dr. Michelle Krenek

Prior to embarking on my Chiropractic journey, I was a high school math teacher, and a basketball and volleyball coach. While teaching at Klein Forest in Houston, Texas, I was involved in a motor vehicle accident: I was at a complete stop and rear-ended by a car going 50 mph. I was taken to the emergency room. After an examination that included x-rays, the doctor told me I was fine. He sent me home with pain medicine and muscle relaxers.

A few months later, I began having headaches, radiating pain down my arm, and severe overall discomfort and fatigue. A friend recommended her chiropractor. Like so many, because I had no experience with Chiropractic, I questioned her on how it would help me—and I went later that year.

A year later, I had my first consultation with Dr. Schels at Advanced Chiropractic in Temple, Texas—and that was the beginning of my life-changing journey. I started seeing Dr. Schels regularly. Soon my pain disappeared, and then I noticed my fatigue slipping away. I felt more energetic, I stopped getting sick, and I even slept better. This is when I knew I had to do more research into this "Chiropractic thing."

In January of 2006, I entered Chiropractic school. In 2009, I opened my first practice in Houston, where I was able to see many patients, host a Saturday morning radio show, and appeared on Great Day Houston once a month to share the miracles of Chiropractic. In 2010, I founded Back To Life Chiropractic in San Antonio, Texas.

Where There is Hope

HOPE ... a feeling of desire for something and confidence in the possibility of its fulfillment.

"Dr. Michelle Krenek was the first doctor to offer me hope for my condition. When I started seeing her, I was taking four medications. Now, I am down to zero and feel like a new person. Thank you, Dr. Krenek, for caring!"

LAUREN C. (twenty-five years old)

Hope is one of the most powerful emotions we possess. Most people I meet, in and out of the office, have such little hope. They accept their lives as they are and never realize that they could actually live at 100 percent of their potential. Patients' believing in their own healing and in their bodies' ability to heal itself, and my convictions and confidence as their chiropractor are all important factors in patients getting well. The most effective way for people to gain faith in their healing is to have confidence in Chiropractic—the doctor and the office.

My belief and convictions about the benefits of Chiropractic care have gotten stronger with every patient I have had the honor to work with. My passion burns so brightly that when I share the value of Chiropractic, there is no doubt in my patients' minds. They can see and feel my heart through my words.

Many people will hear stories about Chiropractic; many will doubt Chiropractic; yet few will ever experience the life-changing power of Chiropractic. My goal, as a chiropractor, is to reach those people who do not know the truth; and to help them see and experience their full potential. (I also want to encourage Chiropractic students through my experiences to strive to discover and live their purpose and to develop their faith, confidence, and belief in Chiropractic so they too can impact the world.)

Our mission at Back To Life is to make sure every person we come in contact with hears the story and realizes why having Chiropractic in their life is a vital part of living to their fullest potential. We know that every person we affect will share their experience with their friends and family, and it is our goal to make their Chiropractic experience exceptional. Each person will experience Chiropractic in his or her own way.

The best way to create great results is to be open to new possibilities, and trust in the doctor and in your body's ability to be well.

I was not confident in Chiropractic until it affected me personally. At that moment of discovery and transformation, I knew I wanted everyone to experience the value that I had experienced. I wanted that blessing for humanity. While in school, I worked hard academically and strove to learn every bit of information I could from the books, my teachers, and my mentors. During this time, I searched for difficult cases so I could see how Chiropractic could help people who had been told something was unfixable. Many people I met lived in misery. They had accepted that state as their life, their cross to bear, because someone told them it was their fate.

I went into every doctor/patient interaction with optimism. I shared what I knew scientifically about how Chiropractic could change their life and health in positive ways. I conducted the necessary examinations and interventions and created care plans; and then let their bodies do the healing. I assured my patients I could help, because I knew without a doubt they would benefit from Chiropractic. With confidence that they would respond in some way, hope and faith in their bodies was gained, and these patients knew that one day they could be normal again.

While a student, we conducted a case study on one of my patients. As a group, we chose this particular patient because a positive response to Chiropractic was not expected. For years this woman suffered with serious discomfort. She had a constant irritation on her back, and always felt the need to scratch. She had been doing this for so long that she developed a scar over the area. An examination revealed that Chiropractic would be of value in helping her complaint of low-back pain.

We started adjusting her with this in mind, not expecting results concerning the itching, even though I must admit I was somewhat hopeful. I understood the power of an adjustment, but still was not fully confident in my expectations or my expression of them. The patient's pain quickly subsided and she was able to move better than she had in a long time. With trepidation, I asked her about the itching. I understood the power of the nervous system, and recognized that the possibilities were endless. I was elated when she shared that her urgency to scratch subsided to the point where she no longer felt it at all. We were even amazed when her scar slowly healed. As a student intern in the outpatient clinic, I had just witnessed something I deemed to be my first miracle as a chiropractor. This woman had been told she would have to live with a nagging condition for the rest of her life—yet with Chiropractic, her life was restored.

I took two lessons from this experience. It is not up to me to decide whether a patient will or will not get better. And who am I to doubt the power that made the body can heal the body? I realized my task is to analyze patients to detect whether or not they have nervous-system interference; and when appropriate, deliver a Chiropractic adjustment and let their bodies do what they can to heal. The other lesson I learned was that a lack of hope, along with chronic pain, can affect someone's life significantly. The misery that comes with the hopelessness that you might never get better can ruin your life.

This experience sparked my faith in Chiropractic. With every miracle I witnessed, my faith, confidence, and belief in the human body and Chiropractic increased.

During this period of time, at an all-school Wednesday assembly, one of my mentors shared a story of a traumatic injury his son Christopher experienced as a teenager. Dr. LaMarche described how during this crisis, even after two decades of being a chiropractor, he did not think about adjusting his son. Dr. LaMarche told the story about the night of July 1, 1999; that he remembers ever so clearly. He, Christopher, and Christopher's friend Matthew were at the LaMarche's lake house. It was time for Dr. LaMarche to go to bed; so he told the boys to be sure to put out the campfire and stay away from the lake. Shortly afterward, two loud booms awakened Dr. LaMarche, but he went back to sleep thinking it was just fireworks for Canada Day. On the third boom he awoke; not because it was loud but because he heard his son screaming, "Help! I can't see!"

Dr. LaMarche jumped out of bed and ran the eighty-eight steps to the lake front. He saw Christopher standing, frozen, with flames coming off his face. He grabbed Christopher by the seat of his pants and the scruff of his neck and dipped his son's face in the lake water; then he carried him up to the house, wrapped his face in ice, and rushed him to the hospital. Christopher was blind in both eyes and had second- and third-degree burns on more than 50 percent of his face. (Christopher, having read that the cartridge contained two blasts, bent over to pick it up to dip it in the lake for safety reasons. Unfortunately, there was a third blast which stuck him in the face, burning his nostrils, his soft palate, and his sinuses. He had no eyelashes or eyebrows left.

When Christopher got to hospital he asked for three things: his brother and sister, the same medication they gave him for pain when he broke his arm the year before, and an adjustment. Through all this, Dr. LaMarche says he had not even thought to adjust Christopher's spine, but he did.

The doctor said Christopher's eyes were burnt 50 percent into the vitreous and the prognosis was likely blindness for the rest of his life. They then flew Christopher to Toronto's Sick Children's Hospital, where they met with two ophthalmologists and three plastic surgeons. The prognosis for his sight was no better. As for the facial burns, the plastic surgeons were encouraging and suggested that after a few surgeries he should recover. They did not want to keep Christopher in the hospital because the risk of infection was high, and this would interfere with the plastic surgeries.

So Dr. LaMarche took him to a hotel. The first thing he did was untuck the sheet at the end of the bed and put Christopher in the bed that way so he had access to his neck. He was heavily medicated and sleeping eighteen or more hours a day. Dr. LaMarche constantly checked his atlas to make sure it was where it was supposed to be so his immune system would be highly functioning in preparation for surgery.

On Wednesday, Christopher woke up and asked his dad if he was wearing a blue shirt; he was. That night, Christopher watched an entire movie and could see it. Even being a chiropractor for so long, Dr. LaMarche was still amazed Christopher could see. He continued to adjust him and that next Monday, they went back to the hospital to find out that Christopher had 20/20 vision. The plastic surgeon came in and said, "Oh, my gosh. What have you done to him? Look, he has perfect epithelial cells growing." She called her team in saying, "Look at this! He's not going to need any surgery!"

Dr. LaMarche's goals in adjusting Christopher were to keep him free from infection and to keep his nervous system functioning at its best to prevent any major complications with surgery. What he and Christopher experienced was obviously something totally different!

The miracle of healing is within each of us. The power that made the body heals the body. It was amazing to me, because Christopher had such faith in the power of the Chiropractic adjustment and in his body's Innate ability to heal. His body did exactly what it was supposed to do: heal.

I never forgot that story and it was stories like those that made me search more and more.

I graduated four and a half years ago, and even before that day, I knew without a doubt that I could change the world even if it was one person at a time. As the years pass, I realize that when you can ignite hope in someone's heart and mind, the healing has already begun. That is why Back To Life's slogan is "Expect A Miracle."

"It wasn't what they did ... it was our partnership ... in desire and intention ... that made the healing happen. I also believe the quality of heart energy and presence are factors that elevate the difference in transforming skill and practice into a true service. One can go through the motions but if the heart feels untouched, efforts are about as effective as applying a flame to old charcoal without the boost of lighter fluid. The same goes with presence. Presence of doing good can be good and even great ... one's Presence of Being is what creates the magic and all the miracles!"

This is a beautiful description of a patient's experience. Our goal is to tell the truth and stimulate the hope that people possess but might have lost. I want to share some of the miracles we have seen in our office because I know that whether you are reading this as a potential patient or as a student, what I am about to share will motivate you to search, grow, and discover more.

A male patient in his sixties came into the office complaining of some aches and pains, but more importantly, he was gravely concerned about his left eye. About a month prior, upon awakening, he noticed his left eye was deviated away from the midline and directed toward the left side of his body. He had suffered no trauma that he could remember, and yet he could not control his eye and his vision was affected. He went to multiple doctors looking for answers. None of the treatments for a variety of diagnoses helped his eye. He tried multiple medications, including steroids, but nothing seemed to help.

I remember his first visit to Back To Life. His spirit was amazing. He had never been to a chiropractor and we were his last resort. He initially attended for a consult and a massage. He admitted later he was skeptical and not sure that Chiropractic could help. During our first consultation, I educated him on Chiropractic philosophy, but did not attempt to offer a diagnosis or give him a list of conditions or pathologies. He had heard all of them before with no success. I did say, "I believe we can help you;" and everything in his demeanor changed. He later told me that because he could see I cared about him, and I believed so strongly that I could help him, that for the first time in months he was encouraged. During every visit, we conducted tests to monitor his progress, and every visit his eye and his vision improved. In short order, his eye returned to its normal position.

Of course, we discussed physiology and the scientific aspects related to human function—but to this man, what occurred he deemed a miracle, as did we. We always give credit to the amazing power of an adjustment and the human body's Innate capacity to heal.

I learned very quickly, especially when dealing with people who had lost hope, that they did not need to hear a list of hard-to-pronounce diagnoses. They wanted to know what was causing their problem, whether or not they could be helped, and what hope we had for them; not all the "things" they had wrong.

The next story is about a female in her early twenties who was recently diagnosed with gastroenteritis and put on a lifelong prescription of four different medications. She had been to countless doctors, provided with multiple diagnoses, and was resolved that this was something she would have to live with for the rest of her life. She was a scientist and an inventor, and both her parents were doctors, so she was knowledgeable. Even though a patient who had experienced a "Chiropractic miracle" referred her to us, she came in with little hope of getting better. Her lack of knowledge and experience about Chiropractic kept her a little reserved. During her consultation, she told me of her constant nausea, dizziness, headaches, stomach pain, acid reflux, vomiting, and hot flashes. She related a recent incident when she ate pizza. Her pain was so intense that she felt the need to go to the emergency room. She stated, "Every morning when I wake up I have blood on my lips because at night the acid comes up and burns me inside." My response was, "I can help."

Sometimes people are a little surprised when they hear my words, but this is something I have complete confidence in. I do not tell them exactly what might happen or what symptoms may subside, but without a doubt I know a Chiropractic adjustment will help them. I believe that this is what they need to hear. I find the subluxation and deliver that adjustment with faith, confidence, and belief—and the healing begins. This young lady's care was very intense, but slowly everything got better. Her nausea subsided, along with her dizziness. Her acid reflux lessened and eventually went away. Her vomiting and stomach pain disappeared. All of her symptoms went away and, more importantly, her body healed. She is now a happy and healthy young lady who experienced a miracle through Chiropractic that has forever changed her future.

In our office, even though we see patients of all ages, we attract a large population of newborns and young adults, a wonderful group to share Chiropractic with. Lately, we are seeing a major increase in the amount of medications prescribed to the younger population, a state that is very disconcerting.

Recently a one-year-old was referred to our office. She had suffered from acid reflux from the time she was a few weeks old and was on a daily regimen of medication since the diagnosis was rendered. In addition, her mother told me that the child got fussy every evening and had trouble sleeping at night. She also said that her child appeared uncomfortable all the time. She was constantly moving and stretching her body. After the first adjustment, there was almost an immediate response. Her mom stated, "I could tell things were changing on the inside, even on our way home." After a few visits, we saw a difference in her personality and an apparent decrease in the symptoms she had been experiencing. The toddler is now off all medication, and she is a happy, healthy baby with a perfectly functioning nervous system—for the first time since her birth.

The next patient injured herself when she and her friends flipped the golf cart they were in shortly after her senior year in high school. She walked away from the accident but later that night was unable to move her lower limbs. She was rushed to the emergency room and diagnosed with a fractured L2 vertebra and immediately taken to surgery. Since that surgery, she experienced burning and tingling in her left leg almost daily. When in the sun for more than ten minutes her left leg would become discolored and painful. She was discouraged at the thought that she had to live with these symptoms for the rest of her life. Having never been to a chiropractor, she decided to "give it a try" with little expectation of any positive response. We monitored her time in the sun, and even after her first adjustment, the discoloration lessened. The decrease in pain was also quickly evident. As she continued to get adjusted, her symptoms slowly dissolved. Today she has no symptoms and feels like a normal twenty-four-year-old.

The last patient I will discuss is a female in her late twenties who came in complaining of neck pain, headaches, and allergies. As we do with all of our patients, we shared the Chiropractic story, how and why Chiropractic works. During the consultation, she revealed that she and her husband had been trying to get pregnant for a year and a half with no success. I shared with her the success rate of Chiropractic care and fertility, and also gave her hope that once her body began to function as it was designed, her chances of becoming pregnant would increase tremendously. She started getting regular adjustments and her pain and symptoms quickly subsided. A month or so after her first adjustment, she walked into the office with an unmistakable glow. She found out the night before that she was pregnant. Since then, we treated her husband, who had daily discomfort with numbness and tingling in his leg and foot for years. He has fully recovered. Now, they come in for maintenance care, and even "our little baby" knows when he/she is at the chiropractor. I can simply lay my hand on our client's belly and he/she will respond with an energetic little kick even if he/she has not moved all morning. It is almost as if the baby knows where he/she is and is shouting for joy because Mommy is about to get adjusted. This is one of the most amazing experiences I have ever been blessed to experience as a chiropractor.

I share these stories so you can know that so many lives have been changed for the better through Chiropractic. Once you witness the amazing power of a Chiropractic adjustment firsthand, your life will be forever changed. Even as I write these words, my heart, soul, and being are excited. Once you experience such profound changes, either as a patient or chiropractor, this is a feeling you will always remember, and one that will consistently fuel your passion.

I encourage everyone to share their experiences with the exceptional power of Chiropractic. You never know how far-reaching something you share today will affect the lives of people tomorrow. Please do not miss out on the opportunity to positively affect someone's life. Share your success stories and provide hope to someone who has lost hope in their own healing power, so they can live a happy successful life by choosing a Chiropractic wellness lifestyle. A little smile of hope can change a life.

About the Author

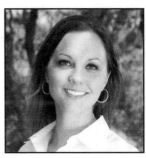

DR. MICHELLE KRENEK graduated from Parker College of Chiropractic in December 2008 and practices in San Antonio, Texas. In high school and college, she was active in all sports, but her passion was basketball. From Fayetteville High School, she went on to play collegiate basketball at Temple Junior College, then at Cameron University. Dr. Krenek graduated from the University of Texas at San Antonio in 2002 with a Bachelor of Science degree in Kinesiology and a K-12 teaching certificate in Physical Education.

As a dedicated chiropractor at Back to Life Chiropractic, she brings hope to people who have lost it. She chooses to inspire people to care about themselves and not depend on drugs as a means of hiding symptoms. Dr. Krenek's health philosophy is simple: when the body can communicate and function at 100%, no feat is impossible. Optimal body communication is accomplished through the Chiropractic adjustment.

Dr. Krenek's passion for Chiropractic is unyielding.

Back To Life Chiropractic is a happy and inviting place. They strive to be encouraging and uplifting for all of their patients because they know that every person who walks through the door has difficulties and challenges. Their office is a place where you can escape from those realities; it is a healing environment where you can focus on yourself and your healing.

Where there is hope THERE ARE ENDLESS POSSIBILITIES.

To schedule an appointment for you and your family, or to book Dr. Krenek to speak at your workplace, church, or civic organization, please visit her website: www.backtolifesa.com.

You can also contact Dr. Krenek at:

Back To Life Chiropractic
1370 Pantheon Way, Suite 160
San Antonio, TX 78232
Phone: (210) 494-3000
Email: drkrenek@gmail.com

CHAPTER FOUR

Tiny Adjustments ...
Great Expectations

Dr. Devin Jeanne Vrana

Pediatric health trends suggest there is a strong possibility that this generation of children could be the first in history that may not be healthy enough to outlive their parents.

- *1 in 6 children has a learning disability or developmental delays*[1]
- *1 in 9 children suffers from asthma*[2]
- *1 in 10 children struggle with ADHD*[3]
- *1 in 50 children develop some degree of autism*[4]
- *1 in 400 children will become diabetic*[5]

One third of children are overweight or obese. Obesity rates have doubled in children and tripled in adolescents in the last thirty years.[6,7]

> All kids need is a little help, a little hope,
> and someone who believes in them.
>
> MAGIC JOHNSON

Look around. The above-mentioned facts are only the tip of the iceberg! Over the past few decades, we have seen increases in illness, disability, and disease in our children by two, four, even tenfold! Our children are sick and they are suffering. The writing is on the wall. Something has gone terribly awry.

But wait, children are supposed to be healthy, right? How can this be happening? Unfortunately, the health trends reflect the very real and eminent future that WE are creating for our children.

---

1. Boyle CA, Boulet S et al. Trends in the Prevalence of Developmental Disabilities in U.S. Children 1997-2000. *Pediatrics* 2011.

2. Schwartz A, Cohen S. ADHD Seen in 11% of U.S. Children As Diagnoses Rise. *The New York Times* March 31, 2013.

Modern medicine continues to push the envelope with technological breakthroughs and medical concoctions. The Internet has given us round-the-clock access to health information—true *and* false—more data than we could ever know how to sort through and comprehend. The United States is the wealthiest country per capita in the world. Shouldn't it also be the healthiest? The sad fact is that the United States is nowhere near the top of the list of healthiest countries worldwide. In fact, when the World Health Organization (WHO) analyzed the overall health status of all countries, the United States fell short, to say the least. Their study ranked the U.S. at #37. I refuse to accept that 37 is the best we can do. I refuse to sit by and apathetically watch the sad state of health affairs in our country. As for the hypothesis that this generation will not outlive their parents—not on my watch!

The purpose of this book is to begin a discussion about how to create a healthier lifestyle. I am a chiropractor who specializes in pediatric and prenatal Chiropractic. (I am also the proud mother of three amazing sons.) I have spent countless hours in lectures and in classrooms—listening, reading, and studying anything and everything I can get my hands on that will help me become a better mother and better chiropractor. I am on a mission and in constant pursuit of truth. I propose that our best bet to have a shot at making a lasting and positive effect on the health status of our country is to start at the very beginning ... with our most-prized possessions: our babies and children.

I believe that *The ART of Being Healthy* begins with the lessons we teach children. Young children have a special light and pureness unlike anything else this world has to offer! While we adults buzz busily through our days, going a hundred miles an hour in a million different directions, children stay present in the moment. They come alive with each new encounter. Children see wonder and true beauty in a way that most adults become blind to as we join "the real world."

Have you ever noticed that special energy of a baby or child? Why are we so drawn to them? We ooh and ahh over newborns. We stare in amazement as toddlers begin to crawl and walk. We cannot help

3. Centers for Disease Control. Blumberg SJ, Bramlett MD et al. Changes in Prevalence of Parent-reported Autism Spectrum Disorder in School-Aged U.S. Children: 2007 to 2011-2012. *National Health Statistics Reports* March 20, 2013.
4. Centers for Disease Control. Asthma Morbidity (U.S.) National Center for Health Statistics Jan. 11, 2013.
5. American Diabetes Association. *National Diabetes Fact Sheet* Jan. 26, 2011.
6. Ogden CL, Carroll MD, Kit BK, Flegal KM. Prevalence of obesity and trends in body mass index among U.S. children and adolescents, 1999-2010. *Journal of the American Medical Association* 2012;307(5):483-490.
7. National Center for Health Statistics. Health, United States, 2011: With Special Features on Socioeconomic Status and Health. Hyattsville, MD; U.S. Department of Health and Human Services; 2012.

but smile when we hear a child laugh. And their tiny gestures of love and innocence can knock us to our knees in a split second. Children embrace life with eyes, arms, and hearts wide open.

Do you remember what it was like to be a child—to be filled with that special magic? I believe adults are drawn to babies and children because the best parts of ourselves long to find a way to get that special something back into our own hearts and lives. Have you taken a long look at children lately? Are we making the right choices for their health and wellness? What legacy are we creating for their future?

I call out an S.O.S. to parents, teachers, families, friends, and health care practitioners of all disciplines. I say ENOUGH with the projected doom and gloom ahead for our children! I say NO MORE turning a blind eye to the path we are laying down for our children! I say NOW is the time for real discussions and serious action! Let's grab the reins and steer this ship in a direction of hope and prosperity.

First, let's talk about what is making our children sicker than they've ever been. Then, let's discuss a game plan for the future. Ultimately, we will see that making *tiny adjustments* today will unlock better tomorrows for our children and us.

What's Going On?

To find a solution to the current health crisis, the focus must shift from *symptoms* to finding the *root cause*. That means that to understand the health of America's children, we must first see the world through the state of stress they are forced to deal with on a day-to-day basis. From the moment a baby is born, a variety of stressors await him or her. We cannot eliminate stress in our children's lives, but we can make an honest effort to understand it better. Building a healthier future for our children starts with seeing the physical, chemical, and emotional stresses they face along their journey.

Physical Stress
Our Children are in Pain

Birth trauma, learning to walk, athletics ... oh my! I challenge you to study the amount of physical stress our babies and children undergo. Look at how babies are being born and the amount of physical stress that is placed on their fragile bodies. Look at the physical stress toddlers and children endure as they learn new motor skills like walking, jumping, climbing, and riding a bike. Look at how youth athletics has changed—increased contact, competition, and commitment demanded in year-round sports of all kinds—at much younger ages than only a few decades ago. Falls and trauma, bumps and bruises inevitably await our babies, toddlers, and children. Luckily, the human body was perfectly designed for such a physically demanding learning process. Children are amazingly resilient, but stress does accumulate. Unless we protect and support our children through these changes and demands, stress adds up and begins to take a toll with long-lasting effects a child will live with for years.

Let's begin our discussion with babies. For nine months, the baby develops in the protection of a mother's womb, completely dependent and at the mercy of her health choices. Hopefully, the mother does the best she can to create a safe, nurturing environment for her developing child. However, even under the most ideal of circumstances, there will be stressors on mom and baby. The baby will carry the effects of that stress into the world.

This brings us to labor and delivery. Most women will tell you that while their child's BIRTHday is beautiful and amazing, the birthing process can be extremely stressful and difficult. I think we can all agree that birth is not an easy process for mom or baby. Even under the best experience, birth can be traumatic. In cases where birth interventions occur, the level of physical stress on the baby increases significantly. The use of forceps, vacuum, and C-section interventions create a dramatic increase in the amount of torque, pull, and pressure on a newborn's tiny spine, nervous system, and surrounding structures. It is estimated that during a C-section, a force in excess of seventy to ninety pounds of upward pull is applied to the newborn's neck. How comfortable does that sound to you? When trauma to the cervical spine occurs during a forceps-assisted, vacuum-assisted, or C-section birth, pain and dysfunction will surely follow. What happens to babies when they are forced to live with the dysfunction and pain? How can they tell us they are hurting from the birthing process? Most likely, they will cry, fuss, and scream.

Are We Listening?

Almost daily, parents bring babies to our office for evaluation. Many parents look to us desperately for help because their babies seem miserable all the time. Typically, parents are told their baby has colic and there isn't a whole lot that can be done. They hold the babies a certain way, prop them up in bouncers or swings to encourage sleep, quiet the baby with a pacifier, use over-the-counter gas drops or gripe water—but, nothing works.

Not being able to soothe the newborn and having to listen to the painful and constant cries can drive parents and an entire household crazy. Not being able to help when your child is in obvious discomfort is one of the most heart-wrenching things a parent can experience.

Remember when we talked about the trauma associated with birth? Thank goodness for chiropractors who are trained to evaluate for spinal misalignments that occur due to birth trauma. All babies should have their spines checked and adjusted, when necessary, to remove the physical stress on their little bodies. Gentle, tiny adjustments allow babies to comfortably unwind after the birthing process. Let's move on to learning motor skill milestones like rolling over, crawling, walking, running, and jumping. Neurologically and developmentally, the first year of life is the most active and important for a child. Physical stress on the baby during the motor development process can be significant. We do not always help them out. Long durations at inclines in car seats, bouncers, swings, and walkers place excessive stress on babies' spines and surrounding structures before they have the strength to support the weight in those positions.

Think of when you've learned a new activity. Oftentimes you will be sore from using muscles you hadn't used in a while. Or sometimes it feels as though there is a kink in the chain because of forces from the new activity. Adults are not the only ones who feel soreness. Consider how quickly a baby develops and a child changes. Surely, you can see how children can become uncomfortable in the process. Proper support is absolutely crucial during this time of rapid growth.

Children also undergo additional physical stresses as they become older. Heavy book bags, video games, cell phones, and sports are a few of the heavy hitters on. Does your child know how to properly wear a book bag? Do YOU know how to properly wear a book bag? Uneven distribution of heavy weight on a child's back can create muscle imbalances and a host of postural compensations. Eventually, your child's spine will adapt. This is just one contributing factor that leads to postural abnormalities and/or spinal curvatures.

Technology has created a bit of a monster for our children. Did you know that there is actually a diagnosis for what is being called "text neck?" From video games to texting and using smart phones, children are glued to handheld devices which is creating a real pain in the neck. Now, I am not proposing that we take all of these things away. But watch them closer. Muscle memory is a powerful thing. We are what we repeatedly do. If a child spends too much time on a device or playing video games, he or she will eventually begin to keep that forward head posture. This will lead to pain, headaches, and postural shifts. Pay attention. Enforce rules and regular breaks from the devices. Do your best to avoid allowing extended periods of play or dependency throughout the day. All you can do is the best you can do, and it all begins with awareness.

Exercise and sports are good for kids—no question! The benefits from regular activity play a crucial role in the optimal development of a child's physical and mental health. But how much is too much?

Youth sports are starting at a younger age. Kids sometimes play multiple sports at a time, year-round, before they even reach middle school. If you ask anyone who played sports in middle school, high school, or college, they will most likely tell you that they suffered some type of injury or carry some level of compensation from the wear and tear they experienced as an athlete. With that said, if we have our children on the field at a younger age, and in a higher level of competition than ever before, we can safely assume that they will grow up carrying greater effects of the wear and tear that will follow them later in life.

Look around and you will notice the effects of physical stress on babies and children. Head tilts and slumped posture, colic and scoliosis, text neck and sports injuries. Our babies are in pain! Our children are a mess! Factor in how rapidly an infant develops and how fast a child grows and changes, and you will begin to acknowledge that there is a constant and demanding amount of physical stress in our babies' and children's lives each and every day.

Have you heard the saying "As the twig is bent, so grows the tree"? The impact of physical stress shapes children for life. Chiropractors are the most educated and qualified to assess your child's spine and nervous system, make necessary adjustments, and support their bodies through this critical developmental process.

Of course I cannot discuss every physical stress that babies and children experience as there are far too many. I do hope that some of the examples get you thinking and paying closer attention than you did before reading this book. Let the process of change begin.

Chemical Stress
Our Children are Sick

What goes in must come out. Junk goes in. Junk comes out. We can apply this concept to the foods that we eat and the medications we ingest. These are dangerous triggers that bring chaos and chemical stress to our internal systems. Short of living in a bubble, avoiding chemical stressors in the environment is impossible. However, knowing what to look for and how to make better choices for you and your family is key.

Food: Junk in the Box

Shall we start with food? It is, after all, the fuel we feed our engine. You have heard the saying "You are what you eat." Do we even know what we are eating or what we are feeding our children anymore? Take a look at the nutritional facts table on the side of a box in your pantry. Can you pronounce all of the ingredients? Is it even food? In the age of genetically modified and highly processed food, our children's digestive systems are under assault on a daily basis. The time has come to get back to basics.

- *Cut the sugar.*
- *Pass on the junk.*
- *Stay away from artificial sweeteners and dyes.*
- *Watch out for reactions to common food allergens (like wheat, dairy, gluten, eggs, peanuts, soy and shellfish).*
- *Shopping at the grocery store needs to be done from the outside aisles. If it can sit on a shelf for weeks or months, do you really want to be eating it? Typically these items fill the interior aisles.*
- *Don't bring the enemy in the house. If you do not bring junk food home, it sure is harder to eat it.*
- *Go for the SUPER foods. Ex: blueberries, sweet potatoes, salmon, spinach, kale, garlic, tomatoes, pineapples, carrots, and water.*
- *Keep it simple and limit portions. We do not need buffets or complex four-course meals. Aim for simple nutritious combinations of real foods that give the body life.*

What about picky eaters? The truth is, your children will eat what you provide them. Be firm. Make good choices, even if it is difficult sometimes. Stick to your guns. You cannot shelter them every single second from bad foods, but you can empower them with the lessons you teach about healthy foods and healthy eating habits.

Food choices and eating habits determine a child's short- and long-term health. Asthma, allergy/sinus, behavioral and focus problems, digestive problems, and obesity are all intricately related to dietary choices. Instead of starting children out addicted to junk, fill their bellies with nutritious foods.

Medication: The Drugging of Our Children

Although the United States makes up only 5% of the world's population, it is estimated that Americans consume 50% of all prescription drugs worldwide—the highest of any country. When I was born in 1983, federal vaccination recommendations were twenty-three doses of seven vaccines between two months and six years of age. Today's vaccination schedule is on a steep climb—sixty-nine doses of sixteen vaccines between the day of birth and age eighteen. Forty-nine of those doses are given before the age of six!![8,9] Sadly, America's children are some of Big Pharma's most regular customers.

8. Centers for Disease Control. Recommended Schedule for Active Immunization of Normal Infants and Children - 1983.
9. Centers for Disease Control. Advisory Committee on Immunization Practices (ACIP) Recommended Immunization Schedule for Persons Aged 0 Through 18 Years – United States, 2013. MMWR 2013; 62(01): 2-8.

Babies come to my office, only days or weeks old, and they have already been prescribed one, two, and sometimes three different medications. A quick poll of a local classroom will reveal that the majority of the students consume at least one over-the-counter or prescription medication on a regular or daily basis. Well-baby visits to the pediatrician for shots have become so mainstreamed, most parents never stop to ask why so many or what is in those vials anyway?

Are there side effects from these meds? You bet! But you will rarely find a commercial that mentions the side effects for over-the-counter and pharmaceutical medications on children. Why? Because it is easier to push a product if you focus on the pros and keep quiet about the cons. Side effects of some of the most commonly used over-the-counter and prescription medications used in pediatrics include: *bloating, abdominal pain, headaches, dizziness, nausea, fatigue.* Are those symptoms that a baby or young child can describe to a parent? Terrifyingly, a baby or child can deal with pain and side effects from a medication for a long time before they are ever caught.

Dependency? Pink potions and magic lil' pills offer a quick fix to symptoms or the temporary illusion of suppression of an illness. My question is: what is the long-term plan? Will the child be required to take the medication to improve function indefinitely? Or, are we looking to just help the child get by for a short term? Children present to their doctor and are diagnosed with a variety of conditions; then they go through a series of trials with different medications and dosages. Eventually, the doctor will get it dialed in and keep the child on a particular drug until they see that the child's physiology has "normalized." So, the child must continue to take that medication indefinitely in order for them to be "healthy."

Seriously?!? Is this our best option? Have we lost our minds? DANGER! Children are being labeled and taught that they are broken or not quite right. Instead of building super-heroes, we smack a label on kids that they will wear for life and usually "need" shots or pills to go with it.

Do the benefits outweigh the risks? Ultimately, no one can make that decision for a parent. The goal of this discussion is not to persuade you to throw away all medications and cease all vaccinations. I have been on both sides of that fence. For the first few years of my first son's life, I did not ask questions. I lay him down for shots and administered medication just as I was told. I would not say that he was a sick child; but he definitely was not a well child. I could see his potential being stunted. The medication was not making him healthier; it was just suppressing his symptoms—often leading to a different health issue. This path led me to begin asking questions.

Now I ask and pose questions in his honor and in the honor of every baby and child I care for. One of my favorite professors in Chiropractic school, Dr. Geracimo Bracho, would often say, "If you don't know, then you don't know." Now that you have become a part of this discussion, you cannot go back. Ask questions about side effects, dosages, frequency, etc. Demand answers. Your child's health depends on it. My challenge to you is to really think before you subject your child's body to any and all types of chemical stressors. You do not have to become anti-medicine; but instead aim to be a responsible, safe, and educated health care decision-maker.

I had the privilege to represent the United States in Beijing, China, at an International Integrative Medicine conference with world-renowned Dr. Richard Yennie and the Acupuncture Society of America. Speakers from all over the world discussed the top health issues and interventions. Medical doctors, surgeons, chiropractors, acupuncturists, Chinese medicine specialists, kinesiologists, PhDs, nutritionists—you name it. There were representatives from every different discipline in health care and background and culture.

One speaker in particular stood out. He was a medical doctor and chaired a prestigious department at one of America's finest colleges. He spoke about the wonders of modern medicine. He discussed the achievements of health care research and development in the United States. Not a soul on earth could discount the genius at our disposal, he said. On the other hand, he spoke of the dangers that accompany the direction our current health care model is headed. As far as acute emergency medicine, there is no doubt that the United States could be considered the best of the best. But for day-to-day health care management of things like the common cold, allergies, infections or aches and pains, we all too often jump to dangerous medications and surgeries before less invasive and highly effective options are considered. This leads to side effects, unnecessary injury, and sometimes death. Currently, when a person of any age becomes ill in our country, the order of care is: (1) medication, (2) surgery, (3) alternative health care options. He proposed that our country could reverse our health trends into a positive direction if we reversed the order: (1) natural health care, (2) medication, (3) surgery.

I could not agree more!

There is a time and a place for medications and surgeries. But labeling a young child, or even worse a newborn, with a condition that leaves them dependent on shots and pills for life CANNOT be our best answer.

Imagine the cost. Imagine the dependency. Imagine the dangers.

CUT the CRAP

If there was a better word, I would use it—but *crap* pretty much sums up our diets and over-medicated sick-care habits in the United States. It is time to think long and hard about what we put in our bodies. What goes in must come out. Good stuff in. Good stuff out!

Emotional Stress

Our Children are Stressed Out

How many times have you told a friend that you've been feeling stressed or that you can feel the tension in your shoulders? We all struggle daily to balance the stressors in our lives. Even the things we enjoy the most bring a certain amount of stress and anxiety to the table. And surely you don't believe that stress is a phenomenon that only adults deal with. Academics, athletics, peer pressure, media, family relationships—those are just some of the things that our young people are bombarded with on a minute-to-minute basis. Not only are a child's stresses real, sadly the child is nowhere close to being fully equipped to deal with all of it.

Do babies experience emotional stress? Of course! They go from being nice and cozy in their mother's womb to loud noises, bright lights, and chaos. They need support, love, and nurturing through that transition. Babies and toddlers change physically at an amazing rate. In and out of cars, introduction to new faces and new places, bonding with siblings, family, and friends are all examples of situations that can be stressful.

Do children and adolescents experience emotional stress? Yup! This is when life starts to get interesting. They stress about discipline, sleep, and health. They long for approval and love. They must learn the harsh lessons of failure and sadness. The world spins faster each and every day.

Perhaps one of the biggest emotional battles children face today is a constant over-stimulation from video games, smart phones, and fast-paced cartoons on television. We live in a world of instant gratification and hyper-stimulation. We allow children to become a part of the madness by giving them access to these devices at very young ages. Even my two-year-old twins come racing to my phone, begging for Mickey Mouse. It is like a drug. The cool noises, the fast movements, and the crazy colors overload their systems and send them racing a million miles per hour. No study has revealed the magic time allotment for TV or video games. In our home, our son knows that an hour of either requires a "fee to pay the toll." Our son knows that to get his game or TV time, he must spend time reading, drawing, doing push-ups, sit-ups, or some form of physical activity. This way, he wins!

Emotional stress brings on a host of health problems: high blood pressure, digestive malfunction, headaches, back pain, concentration and behavior issues, poor sleep, depression, and more. These effects of stress do not kick in after a certain age. They can become a real problem at any age. While adults may turn to a friend or professional to help them deal with stress, children often bottle it up inside. Eventually, their cup will overflow. This is when we see symptoms of illness or disease, self-image issues, changes in behavior and appetite, or even violence. Antidepressants are one of the number one prescribed drugs in the pediatric and adolescent population. These are serious medications with serious side effects. They're crying out for help. Are we really there or are we shutting it down with a pill? It is time to take ownership of our decisions.

Frederick Douglas said, "It is easier to build strong children than to repair broken men." Emotional health is a crucial piece to the puzzle. Pay attention!

Chiropractic

So what the heck does physical, chemical, and emotional stress have to do with Chiropractic?

If I asked ten people why people go to the chiropractor, their responses typically include: *low back pain*, *neck pain*, *injuries*, and *headaches*. While Chiropractic proves to be one of the safest and most effective treatments for those conditions, pain is only the tip of the iceberg of what Chiropractic is really all about.

I have an exercise for you.

Humor me.

Let's begin:

1. **Take your left index finger and point to your brain.**

    This is master control. You know that the brain interprets signals from the body and fires the appropriate responses back. The brain receives all sensory input and controls all necessary motor output.

2. **Take your right index finger and point to your heart.**

    We could choose any organ. But, most people believe that, second to the brain, the heart is our most important organ.

3. **Now, stop. Think.**

    How does your brain communicate with your heart? In a matter of milliseconds, your brain and heart exchange a number of impulses. Muscle contraction, rhythm, rate, etc. You do not have to tell your brain how to communicate with your heart. The nerve impulses fire without you giving them a single thought, and your heart beats as it should.

Let's do another exercise.

1. **Keep your left index finger pointed at your brain.**

   Master control.

2. **Make a fist with your right hand. Open and close your hand.**

   Our hands are our connection to life. They allow us to do so many things, many we never stop to think about (picking up a pen, turning the pages of this book, giving a high-five). The hands serve too many purposes to count.

3. **Now, stop. Think.**

   How does your brain communicate with your hand? In a matter of milliseconds your brain and hand exchange a number of impulses. Muscle contraction, touch, strength, etc. You do not have to tell your brain how to communicate with your hand. The nerve impulses fire without you giving them a single thought.

The brain sends and receives nerve impulses through the nervous system—the brain, spinal cord, and peripheral nerves. Sensory and appropriate response signals are delivered via spinal nerves. The nervous system controls it all.

The nervous system is an important system. We can go weeks without food, days without water, and minutes without air—however, without some nerve impulses, we are dead, instantly. Certainly, it would seem that we would need some protection for a system this crucial to our health and function. The skull and spine are those protectors. The skull protects the brain; the spine forms a bony cage around our spinal cord and nerve exit points. The spine supports and protects the integrity and function of the nervous system.

What happens when stress causes misalignment or dysfunction in the spine? Pressure is placed on the nerve, resulting in alteration of function within the nervous system. When this happens, *the brain CANNOT properly communicate with the structures at the end of the nerve.* Proper communication between the brain and the human body's organs and structures is essential in more ways than most people have ever stopped to ponder.

Chiropractors are trained in the science of locating such misalignments—we call them *subluxations.* Chiropractors are also trained in the art of removing the interference that the misalignment causes within the nervous system. Chiropractors are in fact "nervous system specialists." (The founder and developer of Chiropractic understood the concept of stress and the serious effects it has on human potential.)

Maintaining proper alignment of the spine and promoting proper function of the nervous system is the big picture of Chiropractic.

What Chiropractic Is ...

The vast majority of the population does not understand how or why they would benefit from seeing a chiropractor; and rarely, if ever, would they consider taking their baby or child to get checked and adjusted. While writing this chapter, I realized I couldn't possibly talk about Chiropractic to people who did not understand the science unless I made the effort to see what they see through their eyes. Thus, asked a number of people—patients, parents of patients, family members, friends, and even Chiropractic naysayers what they thought Chiropractic is. For most of them, the response was simple—"Whatever it is doing, it is working. And that is all I need to know."

I then knew this topic merited further discussion. Below I discuss some of the common concerns and misconceptions that I have heard:

• *Once you go to a chiropractor, you have to go all the time—and keep going forever.*
  Well, you don't *have* to go back—but if you find the right chiropractor, you will *want* to go back! Once you experience the positive impact of maintaining spinal alignment and promoting nervous-system health you will not want to stop. You get your hair cut (provided you are not bald) regularly or work out regularly and watch what you eat regularly because you feel better. The same is true for getting regularly adjustments from your chiropractor.

• *I would love to go to the chiropractor, but it is expensive.*
  The issue is not the financial cost; it is that the general population does not understand Chiropractic or the value of an adjustment. I won't go into the ins and outs of the insurance game. Insurance doesn't cover a lot of things in our lives, but that does not deter our need for those things. Ultimately, we all find a way to afford the things that we deem important and necessary. Chiropractic is not cheap. Nothing truly great is—but everything truly great is worth every penny.

• *I don't hurt. Why would I see a chiropractor?*
  Please reference the activity we did earlier when we discussed the communication of your brain to all functions of your body. Chiropractic grew its roots in serving people for things far greater

than pain. You might see a chiropractor for pain, just as you might see a dentist for a cavity or root canal. But you also see a dentist for cleanings and prevention. As you now know, you should see a chiropractor for regular alignments and prevention to improve brain-body communication and maintain optimal function of all systems for a healthy life.

- *Chiropractors pop backs. Is that really necessary and safe for children? Why would a child need to be adjusted?*
Chiropractic is about more than popping backs. It ensures optimal nervous-system function, which is critical to the nerve development and function in all children. No matter the age—hours old or decades old—Chiropractic is necessary and safe. Each adjustment is tailored appropriately to meet the needs of the patient. As far as safety is concerned, Chiropractic malpractice insurance is a fraction of what medical doctors pay. Chiropractors pay less because they have far less probability to harm their patients than medical doctors. Furthermore, research on the safety and efficacy of Chiropractic for babies and children grows daily. I have included links to helpful sites at the end of this chapter.

Unlocking the Power of the Human Potential

Our society is sick. Our society is tired. And, as cliché as it sounds, people are sick and tired of being sick and tired. So, what the heck do we do, folks? WE GET TO WORK!

Imagine a world where children were taught that their bodies could heal themselves. When they skinned a knee, cut a finger, or sprained an ankle, their body heals itself. This Innate healing potential is always present. The appreciation and support of that Innate Intelligence is the key foundation of Chiropractic. B. J. Palmer, dubbed the Developer of Chiropractic, stated, "The body needs no intervention—just no interference."

I propose that health trends for children and adults would improve dramatically and quickly if we could tweak our current health care model. Instead of treating symptoms and managing our health with sick-care, we have an opportunity to shift our thinking to a more holistic, preventative way of taking care of ourselves. The focus must change from suppressing symptoms to locating the cause of dysfunction. Instead of a quick fix", we must start thinking about a long-term wellness plan—support and empowerment of the patient instead of pharmaceutical dependence and invasive intervention.

Our Agreement

Dear Reader,

I will make an agreement with you. I believe that together, you and me—yes, YOU—can begin this crazy journey right now.

I want you to find a picture of a child who is special to you. Go. Find the picture. If that child is near, call his/her name and have him/her sit next to you. I am not going anywhere. I will wait until you are ready.

Ready?

Now, look into the eyes of that child. What do you see?

Beauty?

Sadness?

Innocence?

Stress?

Health?

Sickness?

Obviously, you want the very best for this child, right? You know this child is well worth the investment of your time, energy, and effort to work with them and advocate for them, right?

You are ready to begin the commitment to give them MORE and BETTER, right?

The answers are most certainly YES.

Remember the feeling you just felt.

Long after you have flipped through this book and set it on a shelf with others, I am asking you to remember this feeling.

Hold on to this feeling!!

My promise to you is that I will work each day with that same conviction and love. I will do my part to seek the truth and serve the children and families in my community. I promise to be a leader in my profession so that chiropractors everywhere join me in this promise to you.

Can you promise to do your part by striving to make informed, healthy choices for yourself, that child, and others in your life? Can you promise to be open to natural health care? Can you promise to share this message with your friends and family?

Parenting is not easy. No one is born with all the tools it takes to be a great parent. It is a learning process. We have dozens of tough decisions to make on a day-to-day basis. Connect yourself with local health and wellness experts. Ask for help. Know that you are not alone. Many of the questions you have in your heart at this very instant are questions that weigh on the hearts of parents all around you. The ONLY way that the answers to those questions will ever come to light is if people like YOU begin asking and sharing those questions.

As a wise colleague of mine, Dr. Daniel Rowe, DC, once shared with me, "You cannot change what you do not admit." Friends, it is time to find areas needing improvement, time to admit there is a problem, and time to have the strength to make a change.

The bottom line is that we all need to do the best we can—for ourselves and for those we love the most. Perfection is a figment of our human imagination. The reality is that all we can do is strive each day to do a little better than we did the day before. Magic Johnson said, "All kids need is a little love, a little hope, and someone who believes in them." I believe in them! What if we all began making *tiny adjustments* in our own habits and began making *tiny adjustments* in the lessons we teach our children? Your efforts to empower them will change the destiny of our entire society and planet.

Take this as your challenge to forever impact the health of many, many generations to come!

Yours in the pursuit of health and happiness,

Dr. Devin Jeanne Vrana DC

Resources

Tiny Adjustments: www.tinyadjustments.com

Find a Pediatric Chiropractor: www.icpa4kids.org/
   Find-a-Chiropractor/

International Chiropractic Pediatric Association: www.icpa4kids.org

Mercola Health & Awareness Information: www.mercola.com

National Vaccine Information Center: www.nvic.org

Pathways to Family Wellness Magazine: www.pathwaystofamily
   wellness.org/

Dr. Tim O'Shea Vaccination Research and Resources: www.the
   doctorwithin.com

Well-Adjusted Babies: www.welladjustedbabies.com

~ ~

I dedicate this chapter to my friend and inspiration, Kevin Harp. From a young age, he taught me to be a seeker of truth. Through a variety of health issues, he showed me the power of the human body, mind, and spirit. Because of my friendship with Kevin, my mission is to live a life of service, compassion, and love. My fire is fueled each day by the sound of his voice, "All things are possible. Find what you know to be true and pursue it with your whole heart!"

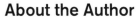

About the Author

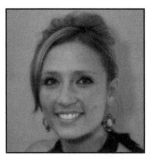

DR. DEVIN JEANNE VRANA is from the heart of America. She grew up in Andale, Kansas—a small town just west of Wichita. In 2006, she graduated with a Bachelor of Science Degree in Kinesiology/Exercise Science from Kansas State University. Dr. Devin went on to earn a Doctorate of Chiropractic degree from Cleveland Chiropractic College. While at CCC, she served as Student Council President, Student American Chiropractic Association Vice President, and Founder/President of the CCC Chapter of the World Congress of Women Chiropractors.

While attending Chiropractic College, Dr. Devin met her husband, Dr. Joey Vrana, DC. The two married just prior to graduation and moved back to their hometown area to open a practice together. After two years in practice, they decided to open a second location to increase accessibility and serve a larger patient base. Dr. Devin and Dr. Joey are committed to working hard to provide safe, all-natural health care to as many men, women, and children as possible.

While both are passionate about the Chiropractic profession and helping people live their best life possible, the Vrana's pride and joy is their three sons—Roman, eight; and twins, Jagger and Knox, two. The Vrana crew loves outdoor adventures, athletics of all kinds, traveling, and family time just relaxing in the backyard.

Dr. Devin loves Chiropractic and helping people—especially babies and children. From newborn to elderly, moms or dads, athletes or weekend warriors, Dr. Devin loves getting to see patients through every stage of life. Dr. Devin has completed pediatric and prenatal specialty training and certification through the International Chiropractic Pediatric Association. She is Webster Technique Certified through the ICPA. Dr. Devin is a Fellow of the Acupuncture Society of America. She has been honored to study and travel alongside Dr. Richard Yennie, pioneer and revered leader in the Chiropractic & Acupuncture professions. She is a member of Pinnacle Chiropractic Management, the Kansas Chiropractic Association, the American Chiropractic Association, EPOC of Wichita, and Junior League of Wichita.

For more information and to reach out to Dr. Vrana, please visit her website: www.backtobasicsChiropractic.net

You can also contact Dr. Devin Jeanne Vrana at:

Back to Basics—Chiropractic and Acupuncture
1247 S. Tyler Road
Wichita, KS 67209
Phone: (316) 440.5554
Email: backtobasics1247@gmail.com

CHAPTER FIVE

The Model of Healthy Living

Dr. Kunal Patel

"Change your thoughts, change your life."

This statement was an eye-opener for me. When you process it, it is undeniably true and can be applied to any part of your life. I encourage each and every one of you to re-evaluate the way you look at everything in your lives, including your health, and what is possible for you.

Take 100% responsibility for your life. If you're not currently where you would like to be in terms of health and well-being, acknowledge that it is due to your actions and poor choices. Once you do that, you gain the power to choose and decide what you're going to do and the direction you will take to create a more fulfilled life. If you blame others or circumstances for the lack of quality and quantity of abundance in your life, then you are living from a disempowered state.

I believe all human beings should be aware of the infinite potential that lies within them. We are truly meant for greatness. There is nothing more valuable than self-work; that is work that you consistently do on growing yourself as a human being. The only person you have the right to judge is yourself. Are you better than you were yesterday? is a question I ask myself every day. To truly live, it is necessary to discover yourself and be on a path of constant transformation to reach higher levels of being. All people who have successful lives are lifelong students of transformation. They are committed to discovering how to constantly become a better version of themselves.

Health is a key component to living a fulfilled life, because when you're healthy, you're able to focus on personal growth and being a valuable asset to others around you. My *why* is simple. I want to help humanity reach its divine potential, to inspire others to focus on themselves, and create the best version of themselves so that as a net result the world can be a more harmonious and supportive place. Health is simple. It boils down to your inner beliefs that dictate the self-respect and value you place on your life. It is my belief that the human body is the greatest temple ever built. It is your true home for your entire life. Very few people do much, if any, work on their bodies and on minds to nourish their higher being. People have become so externalized that they have lost touch with their own self. They have fallen victim to their bodies. It saddens me to see the greatest miracle, the greatest gift that we have been given, abused and neglected.

Create a curiosity to discover how to achieve the best health for you and your family. Inquire about it, read about it, and view informative documentaries about health and healing. The information is available. You have to decide what resonates with you and what seems to be a fad.

I believe that health and wellness are the greatest assets in this world, one that many people don't respect until it's taken from them. Respecting yourself, your body, and the divine wisdom that is always within you. Live proactively. You are responsible for you and very few people care more about you than you care about yourself. You owe it to yourself to be the best version of you possible. In Chinese medicine they say, "Don't dig your well when you're dying of thirst, dig it beforehand." Begin living from a preventative and proactive approach to health so you can live life to the fullest.

One of the greatest tips I can provide you is to create a vision for your life that is much bigger than yourself. Create a vision that ignites you every morning because you know you are living your passion and purpose. When you value your life and have a driving force propelling you, you begin to commit to higher standards for yourself and your family. You snap out of the mind-numbing, unfulfilling acts of going through the motions: waking up, going to work (at a place you may not even care for), coming home, eating, watching TV, going to bed. Everyone has a unique talent, a unique gift created for a higher calling, and a mark to leave on the Earth that will make this planet a better place. You must have this *knowing*, this belief, in order to reach higher levels of living.

You lose the sense of empowerment when you fall victim to institutions that have a vested interest in themselves, in profits, in greed, and power. It is the continued fear that is generated in the media that fuels these vicious cycles of submission and control. It is the collective consciousness of fear that holds us back from achieving all that we were meant for. The health care system in this country is based on fear. There is minimal encouragement and recognition of experiencing optimal health as nature intended.

What I share with you is meant to empower you to take control of your health and your life; to encourage you to discover yourself further; and to embark on a meaningful life filled with lasting joy, peace, and abundance. It is my passion to bring about inspiration and growth to others by way of healthy living for a better world. We are all in it together. We can support one another, uplift one another, and bring positive change.

Define the Art of Being Healthy

The art of being healthy is the masterful creation of an empowered life with continuous expansion into higher expressions of body, mind, and spirit. Health is far more that being pain free, feeling good, and looking good. *Feeling* is a poor indicator of health and low on the spectrum of human potential. Many times people who are the apparent "picture of health" are told they have cancer or heart disease or a multitude of other illnesses that take years to develop. A person can feel good and then one day have a stroke or a heart attack. There is no way that person was healthy. True health is a consequence of optimal *function*, your body working exactly as it is supposed to, not simply the absence of symptoms.

If you only make choices based on how you *feel*, you miss out on the opportunities of discovering vast capabilities that are available to you with a little conscious effort. You can live a life of mediocrity or you can create a masterpiece.

Your life is a work of art. You are the painter, the canvas is the infinite possibility that has been gifted to you, the color of paint reflects your emotional aspect and how you see the world. Since you are the painter, you have the ability and the control to create a life of vibrant art and dimension throughout each stage of your life. And realize, you have been given an infinite supply of blank canvases! Lucky you! At any point in your life, you have the ability to toss the canvas that didn't serve your purpose and begin a new piece of art. As you grow and reach higher levels of being, you are able to build upon your portfolio and learn from previous works to create better, inspiring versions to share with everyone in your life.

Being healthy results from healthy living, which encompasses focusing on key aspects that cumulatively produce a sense of well-being. It is more of a continually applied discipline, a lifelong process, rather than one act or product claiming to make you healthy. It is a puzzle that relies on each piece. Those pieces are: structural integrity of the physical body allowing nerves and vessels to flow unrestricted;

sound mental health, your thoughts, self-talk, the level of respect you hold for yourself; daily acts that bring about spiritual connectedness; uplifting social interactions and relationships; physical fitness, proper whole food nutrition, and purified water, quality rest, and sleep; and minimizing exposure to toxins. If you can bring about small changes in each of these key areas and slowly expand, you will begin to see the amazing things that are possible for you.

A lot of people experience the feeling of a "miracle" when they see a newborn baby. Birth is one of the great miracles of life—but it doesn't stop there. Many people lose that sense of awe about the human body and this magnificent planet that supports us and provides everything we need to live. Instead, we purchase that next fad product or follow that next idea to fulfill ourselves, when in reality all we need for well-being is inside of us. We just need to clear away the dust and cobwebs in our minds that society has helped to establish and realize this truth.

A baby is born with infinite potential, a blank slate ready to create a grand life. But then, this child is molded by its family, by social conditioning, by people who say, "No. You can't do that, you can't have that, you're not deserving." The limiting beliefs of other people get programmed into that baby and the infinite possibilities become greatly reduced for that "once looked at miracle."

I'm here to tell you that you can change that limited way of existing at any time. It is possible. You have to choose and be committed to it. In his books *The Biology of Belief* and *The Honeymoon Effect: The Science of Creating Heaven on Earth*, Dr. Bruce Lipton reveals our ability to re-program our subconscious mind and begin consciously creating the life that we want to live. They both are enlightening and remarkable books that offer insight and scientific truths for empowered living. I encourage you to read them both and start believing in your ability to create the life you dream of.

Like I mentioned earlier, change and growth is a process. Growth in any area takes time. All processes in life take time. Be patient and don't give up on yourself because you are so worth it.

Healthy Habits Should Begin From Birth

It is crucial to instill healthy habits in children at an early age to prevent the buildup of cobwebs and misconceptions that are found in most adults. It is better to create healthy children than fix damaged adults. It is most every parent's desire for their child to live a better life than they live. We want our future generations to be better off than we are. That leads to greater advancement for humanity and better quality of living. The Dalai Lama said, "If every eight-year-old in the world is taught meditation, we will eliminate violence from the world in one generation." Since we cannot control every child in the world, we can focus on our own children and make them the best human beings possible, secure in their ability to create anything they desire, and maybe as adults they will create a system to help contribute to world peace. I urge parents to put into effect systems for empowering their children and supporting their growth. Conventional ways are not always the best and it is up to you to find out from others who have made it their mission to live extraordinary lives.

We live in an extraordinary time when all the ancient wisdom and healing arts are reemerging, at our disposal. This is a time of great change; we can realize truths that have the power to create massive growth for humanity.

Let us take a look at health, and how the body functions.

You Are Your Best Doctor

Chiropractic is based on the foundation of natural laws and the truth that you are your best doctor. It works with and supports the undeniable fact that you have an inborn, magnificent healing capability that no medical doctor can provide. It's irrefutable that there is a genius far greater than anything imaginable that animates and runs your body, for your entire life, without having to think about any of the functions. It takes care of everything for you. Not many people take the time to appreciate this truth and thank their body for all it does. Instead, people expose their body to toxins, abuse, stress, and neglect. Let me remind you: you only get one body. You can either take some steps to support it now, or spend years recuperating your health when serious damage has taken place.

Since many people do not fully understand the far-reaching benefits of Chiropractic care, I will explain what it is in four concise principles:

1. The human body is a self-healing mechanism. If you cut your finger, it heals. If you cut a corpse, it doesn't heal. It is life that heals.

> When asked what surprised him most about humanity, the Dalai Lama said, "Man ... Because he sacrifices his health in order to make money. Then he sacrifices money to recuperate his health. And then he is so anxious about the future that he does not enjoy the present; the result being that he does not live in the present or the future; he lives as if he is never going to die, and then dies having never really lived."

2. The nervous system is the master system of the body. Every dimension of the human experience is governed through the nervous system. Every thought, every action, every motion, every emotion, EVERY element of human life is processed through the nervous system.

3. When there is interference with the function of the nervous system, it compromises your physical well-being and has psycho-emotional implications as well by altering your perception of the world and your ability to respond correctly to your environment.

4. A chiropractor locates and corrects the causes of nervous system interference.

Everything in the Universe is energy and motion. Life is motion. There is a constant rhythm and exchange of energy; this also holds true for our bodies. There is constant birth, growth, and death taking place at a cellular level throughout our lives, all governed by an Innate Intelligence, the same intelligence that created us from two tiny cells. We do not have the same body composition of cells and atoms that we had an hour ago, or last week, or last year; we are constantly renewing. We have the ability to decide if we want the renewal to be for better expression of health and life, or for worse, at any moment by the choices we make every day.

All of this growth and regeneration is regulated by our master control center, the brain. The brain extends down the body as the spinal cord to create a neuronal network that sends and receives information at every level. The spinal cord is the major interstate of transportation of vital messages, energy, and information flow. The vertebral column is the protector of this "super computer's" communication pathway. At each level of the spine, nerves branch out from the neuronal axis at the off-ramp (in between each vertebra), and head to all parts of the body at that level where they innervate and communicate with the various structures of the body.

Things can get backed up at that off-ramp however, and interfere with the flow and exchange of vital communication to and from the brain. When there is a disruption in the flow, energy starts to pool at this region of the body. Optimal life-force energy is restricted, causing a lack of proper message exchange that is vital in regulating body processes. This is known as a *subluxation.*

Wellness chiropractors see the immense value in correcting disruptions in the nervous system (subluxations). Your spine needs to be clear of subluxations for you to be able to reach an expression of health that is ever-expanding.

A subluxation affects the body in five major ways:

1. Kinesiopathology—Spinal joint motion that has become reduced, creating irritation and inflammation of the spinal disc and joints in the region where nerves exit the spinal column.

2. Neuropathophysiology—the aberrant spinal biomechanics produce a whole body response due to inflammation and irritation of delicate nerve tissue. Symptoms are not always obvious because only 10-15% of the nervous system has fibers designated for pain. This is why it's important to get checked even when you are asymptomatic. Many patients experience improvements to health issues that are not usually associated with the back.

3. Myopathology—Muscles that support the spine and your skeletal structure become flaccid and weak, or become tight, going into spasm. It takes time to retrain the muscles and ligaments to regain structural integrity of the spine.

4. Histopathology—Spinal discs, ligaments, and cartilage have a poor blood supply. These tissues depend on the pumping action of joint fluids to supply nutrients and expel waste products. When this pumping action is impaired, these critical soft tissues do not heal with the speed today's patients want or expect. It takes time and consistency to heal and bring about changes to years of abnormal function.

5. Pathophysiology—Over time, if a problem is neglected, the body will attempt to splint or stabilize the injured joints. This is when degenerative changes begin to set in. When this occurs, other tissues and organs are affected due to deprived normal nerve supply.

Since the entire body is connected, when you have hindered function at one area, the whole body is affected and performs less than it is capable of. Who wants a body that functions less than the infinite potential available to it? No one!

You may be wondering how subluxations occur. In one short answer: stress. Stress, whether it's physical, emotional, and/or chemical can cause distortions in the characteristics of the body and lead to inability to adapt. Usually it is a combination of all three types of stress that bring disruptions to the nervous system. Physical stress includes accidents, repetitive falls and injuries while growing or playing sports, strenuous work, poor posture, and lack of exercise. Emotional stress could be worry, anxiety, tension, fear, lack of self-worth, and negativity that create biochemical changes to the physiology and disruption in the nervous system. Chemical stress is from toxins such as cigarette smoke; pollution; additives and preservatives in foods; excess chemicals in beverages, including water; and chemicals put on our skin.

With regular care as indicated by a chiropractor, your body will be able to switch from a defensive state into one of thriving and growth and be better able to adapt to its environment.

Let's face it, stress is a part of life; which is why so many people make Chiropractic a vital part of their family's lifestyle.

Chiropractic adjustments create harmony and balance within the nervous system. It involves a specific force that the body is able to accept and integrate in order to establish structural integrity to the body, thereby allowing for nerve communication to be restored. When the body is in a physiological state of growth and adaptation, your entire being has the ability to evolve and reach higher levels.

> "Quantum physics has found that there is no empty space in the human cell, but it is a teeming, electric-magnetic field of possibility or potential. If we are creating ourselves all the time, then it is never too late to begin creating the bodies we want instead of the ones we mistakenly assume we are stuck with."
>
> DEEPAK CHOPRA

There is no drug or magic pill that's going to make you healthy, so you can throw that belief out the window right now. *Drugs* and the *health* don't even belong in the same sentence or paradigm. What a drug does, a man-made synthesized pill, is try to override the body's Innate Intelligence by taking control of the physiology. Now, I do believe that in emergency situations, your life can be saved by drugs, but to make medication a part of your everyday life is absurd. I know people who are on twelve to fifteen different medications. There is not a single scientist, drug manufacturer, or doctor in the world who can say that a drug interaction of that sort is not harmful to the body. Pills don't have a GPS directing it to the damaged part of the body. Drugs affect the entire system. Leave the quick-fix approach behind, because it does not bring about health. Instead begin on a path, true to you, that supports the function of the body.

Every positive step you take toward supporting your health, whether it's beginning to appreciate yourself a little more, talk yourself up some, adding more vegetables to your diet, spending more time in Nature, getting your spine checked for subluxation—anything that supports your growth and expansion as a human being—is significant and adds to your physiology, adds to your health bank, a bank that only accepts and accumulates healthy actions made by you.

Begin giving the little things more value because they count and are substantial on your path to well-being. Don't put so much pressure on yourself because you haven't been doing *all* the right things that lead to good health. Take a step, then build on it, and soon you'll naturally form the habit of healthy behavior.

The key is to appreciate what you currently do and know that it's a big deal and continue to move in that direction to add more "big deals" into your life. It will be transforming.

Everything is a process and a journey. Take action; work toward base hits. I encourage you to discover yourself, surrender to the unfolding of life, and believe that all things are possible for you.

The Profound Effect of Your Mind

One of the best things you can do for yourself is to take time out every day to be in solitude and focus on you. Whether it's meditating, writing in a journal, visualizing what you want to attract in your life, recalling everything you are grateful for, or purposely creating your life. Alone time is highly nurturing to your mind and spirit. It brings about clarity and relieves stress. Sit in silence and begin masterminding the art that you want to create for your life. Write out your goals in each area of your life. When you have a vision for yourself and a guide to follow, it prevents you from aimlessly going through life, achieving very little of what's available to you.

The mind-body connection is undeniable. Your mind, the way you perceive yourself and your life, affects your physical health and vice versa. I can't emphasize how vital it is to work on mental health every day and the impact it will have on where you "head" in life (pun intended). The way you decide to feel each day will determine how life will flow for you.

Whether you believe it or not, the Law of Attraction is real. What you put your mind and feelings on over a period of time will show up in your life. Negativity and worry attract more negativity and worry. Do away with negative judgments toward anyone as it does not serve your higher being. Dwelling on past challenges and misfortune will attract more misfortune into your life. Everything in life is a lesson. You can both grow and evolve from your experiences and progress on your divine path, or you can choose to be a victim and see the Universe as unsupportive. You can believe that anything is possible for you and you can have whatever you desire, or you can think everyone is out to get you and nothing works out for you. Either way, you're going to be right.

Action Steps

Start and end the day in complete gratitude for everything in your life, along with affirming what you want to create for yourself. Choose to live in a state of gratitude and only focus energy toward what you truly want for yourself. This is a challenge for many people because we have been conditioned into a lack and fear-based mindset; however, with a little work that can be found from self-help books and programs from amazing authors around the world at Hay House and Hay House Radio, your life will begin to take on a new meaning. Believe you can have exceptional health, relationships, and abundance in all areas of your life. Really believe it every day! Don't give up. Most people try it, give up, and then wonder why their life is so poor. The Universe tests you to see how badly you want it and when you wake up each morning unwavering at the new possibilities you have opened yourself up to, you will begin to see it manifest in your life. I promise you, the consistent work on yourself every day, shutting out any negative beliefs about anything or anyone, and only focusing on what you desire will bring about a fulfilling life.

It's your choice to focus on what you want each and every day.

Hydrate your body with plenty of water every day. Choose nutritious foods that support the body. Incorporate healthy fats into your diet and smoothies packed with greens (check out www.foodmatters.tv for great tips on healthy eating). Make a habit of reading the ingredient list on all the products that you buy and eliminate any that you cannot pronounce because chances are they are toxic chemicals. Spend time in Nature, barefoot if possible, and experience all the beauty around you; barefoot because you will draw in the negative ions from the earth, the strongest antioxidant.

Do some sort of physical activity every day, whether it's going for a walk with a significant other or doing yoga, or weight training. Our bodies are made for physical work, beyond desk jobs and sitting in the car on our commute, and lounging at home. Get your heart rate up, get sweating. Start doing activities that you love, that you're passionate about. Get on a consistent sleep schedule and create a peaceful environment in the bedroom that is conducive to quality rest. It is while asleep that your body is actively processing the day's events and bringing out healing and restoration. Proper sleep is crucial to well-being. My last bit of advice is to be around uplifting and inspiring people; people who positively influence your life and growth.

Most importantly, visit a chiropractor and have your spine free of subluxations so that your nervous system is better able to support you in every experience of your life; so you can extract nutrients from your foods efficiently, so your body can coordinate the production of hormones and a physiology that supports you, so you can have muscles firing in correct sequence and integrity to perform work you do with your body, so every organ can function as it is intended to.

The greatest gift you can give your child is to get him or her checked and adjusted for subluxations. Their delicate bodies are growing at such a rapid rate that it is important for their nervous systems to be functioning optimally, even after the traumatic birthing journey. The benefit to their immune system alone is enough for most parents to have their newborn baby checked. As a child learns to stand and walk, small repetitive injuries can add up to dysfunction. There is much information and research available at www.icpa4kids. com as to the effectiveness and importance of Chiropractic care for children.

A Fulfilling, Abundant Life

Commit to a life of excellence—excellence in how you treat yourself; excellence in all of your relationships and how you treat others; excellence in how you see your future; excellence in the way you think, feel, and act; and excellence in how you fuel your body, mind, and spirit. Know that it is never too late to make wise choices. You have the ability to create anything you want with the choices you make. Choose wisely.

Begin putting your newfound knowledge into action, and please share it with others. I believe in your ability to create a magnificent, healthy life.

About the Author

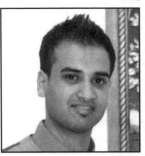

DR. KUNAL PATEL has a vision and belief that by 2025, the United States will be the model for healthy living worldwide; and that now, more than ever before, is an amazing time for change and transition—from systems that lack authenticity and propulsion for human growth to ones that support an ever-expanding advancement for all of human potential.

A December 2012 graduate of Sherman College, Dr. Patel has made it his mission to spread the message of empowered living on a global arena with some of the most amazing people that have inspired him. One of his life goals is to provide support and development to philanthropic causes, such as ending world hunger, initiatives in making sure every human being has clean drinking water, and providing children with higher-consciousness learning.

He is passionate about conveying to people how extraordinary the human body is and the healing power within that is always available. Chiropractic was brought to Dr. Patel by way of a higher calling while he was in undergraduate studies. He had the privilege to meet a remarkable human being, Dr. Kevin Jackson, which lead to an inspiration of human service and empowering others to take charge of their health and ultimately their lives and not fall victim to themselves.

In the last year of Chiropractic school, Dr. Patel began studying and living from the wisdom of some of the current greatest spiritual teachers like Dr. Wayne Dyer, Dr. Bruce Lipton, Louise Hay, and Dr. Deepak Chopra. Dr. Patel's internal state of being, as well as his expression towards life, has shifted and expanded in leaps due to the gift of Chiropractic and a sound mind-body connection, bringing to him a greater sense of peace and joy and the realization of a greater purpose for living which he hopes to inspire in everyone he touches.

For more information, or to invite Dr. Patel to speak at your workplace, church, or civic organization, please visit his website: www.drkunalchiromazing.com

You may also contact him at:

Synchronicity Chiropractic
528 Howell Road
Greenville, SC 29615
Phone: (717) 495-5656
Email: kunalpateldc@gmail.com

*Cherish the past,
embrace the future, and
celebrate life to the fullest
through Chiropractic.*

CHAPTER SIX
Maximizing Health, Performance, and Vitality

Dr. Natalie Bird

I wonder why you chose to read this book. What made you curious and invited you in? Are you currently "healthy" and searching for increased knowledge, answers, and inspiration? Are you struggling with a particular health issue, have tried many forms of treatment, and are at your wit's end with what to do? Are you doing ok with your health, but know you could be doing more and feeling better? Have you heard of Chiropractic, but have no idea what it is all about or how it could possibly help you? Are you looking for a new approach to health care because your intuition tells you there must be a better way? Or, are you already a regular Chiropractic patient who knows and loves the philosophy, who has experienced the difference when your brain and body are connected perfectly, and you are expressing you full magnificence?

Perhaps you didn't choose this book, but it chose you?

Would you like more energy? Would you like to wake up in the morning rested and rejuvenated and excited about what the day will bring? Would you like to feel and function better than you do? Would you like to love the way your body looks, both fully clothed and also when you stand naked in the mirror? Would you like more mental clarity and the ability to cope better with the variety of stressors that life throws your way?

If you answered yes to any of these questions, I'm glad you are reading, and I appreciate your time and trust. Regardless of why, if you want to be healthier, happier, and enjoy life more, you are on the right track.

I am often asked to teach people about true health and vitality, and I want you to know that I feel blessed to be in the position to share with you the things you would find me doing in my home if you popped in for a visit. This is how I live and how my children live.

Being healthy, and respecting and honouring my body is my life. I know that if you take even a small portion of the gems shared in this book, you will come away a better version, the best version, of you!

First, I would like to congratulate you for where you currently are in your health and your life. You have made thousands and thousands of decisions regarding your body, all based on the best knowledge you had at the time. I hope to challenge and excite you to make some positive changes in the way you view your well-being, and I look forward to hearing about them in the future.

I am here to teach you what the pros do to stay healthy. If you want to be rich, do you study rich people or poor people? Likewise, if you want to be healthy, do you study healthy people or sick people? Healthy, for sure!

My expertise lies not only in Chiropractic, but also in how what we *eat* affects how we heal, how our body functions, and how amazing we can be and feel. I am proud to say that my body feels and looks better than it ever has before. I have loads of energy, stable moods and thoughts, great digestion, and I love to exercise in ways that push my body to the limit, making me feel alive and strong.

But, please understand, I am human, and it was not always this way. There was a time when the way I lived did not support a wonderfully vibrant body or a natural, vital approach to health care. I was raised in a beautiful family in Melbourne, with strong family values and bountiful love. We were very much a normal family who played by the rules of society with regard to diet, exercise, and health care choices. My mother made the majority of decisions regarding our health and she was brilliant, she always held our needs before hers and followed the advice of our family medical doctors with unwavering commitment, dedication, and love.

I suffered with severe asthma as a child. I remember being trialled on countless steroid drugs, inhalers, sprays, liquids, capsules, tablets, sprinkles, lotions, potions—you name it. I can't tell you how many courses of antibiotics I have been on or how many times I was an emergency at the local medical practice or hospital. What I *can* tell you is that the feeling of not being able to breathe never ever leaves your memory. Tears well up in my eyes as I write this even now, more than twenty-five years later, recalling the feeling of being a helpless, innocent child, struggling with the basic human requirement of fresh air. I can instantly recall the feeling of my throat tightening, closing over; my lungs heavy, constricted, and compressed. I remember trying desperately to breathe in life-giving oxygen but having nowhere for it to go. I can also recall the terror in my mother's eyes as she looked on in fear as the doctors tried to calm me and medicate me further. It is only now, as an adult, as a mother, that I can begin to understand what she must have gone through, how she must have felt let down, perhaps a failure, after having followed all the advice given to her to manage my health to no avail.

> "Doing the same thing over and over again and expecting a different result is the definition of insanity."
> ALBERT EINSTEIN

I am certain that sometimes, due to the lack of oxygen, I surely would have died without medical intervention. But, I am also certain that if my parents had been led down a different path, if they had been educated from a holistic, vital paradigm of health, then things would have been different. If only they had been taught about the amazing inborn healing ability of the body, a body that is self-healing, self-regulating, and self-organizing. If only there had been someone with a strong enough belief and conviction in the power of the human body, someone who was willing to stand up and be a louder voice than the disempowering ones and teach of an alternate way. If only my mother could have read a book like this and then connected with a community of like-minded families to share support, information, and resources and learn how to approach health from a different perspective. Who knows how different, how much easier, how less stressful my health journey could have been? I promised myself that when I became a mother, I would be armed with the information to make informed decisions about my children's health and do my best to prevent my children ever feeling the way I did, and avoid feeling the way my mother must have.

I am so proud—but also deeply saddened—that my children, ages four and seven, know more about health and well-being than many adults. They see their friends and the ways they eat, drink, and behave, and often remark on how many days of school their friends miss. My children notice that other mothers treat their children as weak and vulnerable, and give them medications to make them better.

Our thoughts, beliefs, and attitudes begin in childhood, and often determine how we see life as an adult. If we are teaching children that health comes from the outside, and that we need to take drugs, remedies, have injections, surgeries, or any other treatments to heal us, it teaches them to always look outside for help. This disconnects people from their Innate Intelligence and from themselves, not only as a self-healing organism, but as a whole person equipped with every tool needed to be exponentially happy and healthy. The outside-in belief system leads you to believe that you are imperfect and ill-equipped for life on every level. This leaves no space for expressing your full potential if you are expending energy fighting off disease and sickness.

It is our role not only to provide our children with the resources to stay healthy but to also instill in them the wisdom that they must respect, recognize, and support their internal power in all its magnificence.

Hippocrates said, "Everyone has a doctor in him or her; we just have to help it in its work.

Kids raised in a Chiropractic wellness lifestyle grow up understanding that we all have within us everything we need to be completely healthy. Our bodies know exactly how to run, regulate, grow, heal, and flourish—everything necessary to express full life. People who live a Chiropractic wellness lifestyle understand that they are perfect and if they look after their bodies, they will be their best. "Looking after your body" means eating foods that Nature made (and supplementing where necessary to ensure your body has all the right building blocks), drinking clean water, exercising, sleeping enough, and at appropriate times, keeping your nervous system switched on, and most importantly giving and receiving loads of love from family and friends. This recipe has empowered my children to trust in their bodies. They know to look inside for health, not outside, and understand they must focus their attention on what they want, not what they don't want. They do not waste time thinking about, or fearing, ill-health, but instead put all their energy and time into promoting great health and vitality. And, believe it or not, it is actually fun!!

We love family challenges of who can run the fastest, who can hold a plank the longest, who can swim underwater the longest. They love seeing how many foods that our body loves they can name, and then foods that make our bodies scream when we eat them. They look forward to their weekly Chiropractic check-ups, and when asked why they get adjusted, they will tell you: "So I can be the healthiest in the world ... so I can be my best ... to keep me healthy!"

We have created a family ritual around the dinner table each night taking turns to describe first our failures for the day and acknowledging what we learned from these, and then what made us smile, laugh, or express love. We praise each other for using words that build ourselves and others up and have a list of positive words that describe the person that we are, and that we are striving to be, and we read this list often. We all have written goals too, even my children. We have developed our own culture that we accept is quite different from many families, in that we don't buy into sickness or disease, but thank our bodies each day for the amazing jobs they are doing, and love and accept any "health expression" (cold or flu, vomiting or diarrhea) that we may infrequently have as a sign that all is well and that our immune systems are in fact working well.

Since 1895, when it was founded, Chiropractic has always been about the body's ability to interpret messages to and from the nervous system. Any interruption to this information highway is called a *subluxation*, which interferes with the nerve signals and reduces our ability to function at 100%. Chiropractor's find these "traffic jams" and correct them; it's as simple as that.

I am constantly in awe of my elderly clients who continue to dazzle and baffle their aging friends with their energy, grace, and flexibility. I see my elite sports people excelling, injury free and at the top of their game. I am so humbled by the power of the body to give back all that you invest. Outstanding health is actually easy to achieve and express with the right action plan, thoughts, effort, and time. This leads me to what I'd also love to share with you, and that is about what you are eating ...

Without a healthy nerve supply to and from your digestive system, you cannot digest, assimilate, and absorb all the nutrition from the food you eat. If you are not eating the right foods, those that we are genetically programmed to eat, you cannot express full health either. Your body is designed to be spectacular! I have noticed overs the years, working with my patients, that there is a lot of misguided fear, guilt, and confusion with regard to what we should be eating and why. Sadly, humans have become the world's sickest animal species. Most eat, drink, and live in ways that are totally unnatural and incongruent with the needs of our cells. We are the only species on Earth that has created a completely unnatural diet and living environment for ourselves. With the right guidance and knowledge, we can re-learn what to eat to maximize our performance. First however, some deeply ingrained beliefs and attitudes must be challenged and overcome. The biggest area this relates to in our diet is our relationship with FAT.

If you are anything like me, I spent at least twenty years on a low-fat diet, trying to keep my body lean and what I thought meant healthy. Countless hours were wasted counting calories, reading food labels, and believing marketing statements on so-called trusted products. What I now know implicitly is that we actually need fat, and lots of it! If you are going to activate your health with the best fuels available, you need to make peace with fat. Contrary to popular belief, eating fat will not make you fat. Fat is critical for human life. For many people, it is hard to let go of the deeply ingrained mistruths that tell us fat is bad. Even now, when I consume loads of fat each day, putting a slab into my daily coffee with one or two tablespoons of coconut oil, I sometimes catch myself thinking, *Gee, that's a lot of fat. Maybe I shouldn't ...* before I come to my senses and remember to delete, delete, delete.

Despite the low-fat craze society has forced on the culture, fat is a normal and essential nutrient in the human diet. Fat is the structural component that makes up your brain and nervous system and most of your endocrine (hormone) system. Together these two systems are primarily responsible for regulating the entire body. Fat is required to absorb vitamins from food, it is used for energy, it is stored for release when more energy is needed, and it is also a major component of the walls in all of our 100 trillion or so cells.

Can I trust you with my secret? Ok, here goes ... I ensure that every meal I consume has a generous amount of fat in it to feed my brain, give me energy, and nourish all my body's systems. My favorite source of fat is organic virgin coconut oil; it is the only oil I cook with. I consume it with most meals, in some way, shape, or form. My breakfast often involves eggs either fried, scrambled, or in an omelet, cooked in coconut oil, or a delicious smoothie of coconut milk, coconut oil, spinach or kale, two raw eggs, berries, LSA meal, raw cacao, and a dash of cinnamon. I usually have raw nut balls of varying ingredients in the fridge that I will have if I need a quick breakfast or a snack throughout the day. With my breakfast, I take more fat in a fish oil supplement to maximize my brain power and ensure I am completely full of fat to fuel my day. In the summer, my lunch is usually a salad with walnuts, sunflower and pumpkin seeds, avocado, and generous slurps of olive oil; in winter, I have soup cooked with coconut oil and bone broth that has drawn out all the good fats and nutrients from the meat or chicken bones. My evening meal will generally be a roast, stew, or barbecued meat, always grass-fed, free-range, and organic whenever possible. I definitely enjoy eating the fat and skin too, understanding that it will provide my body with essential building blocks for repair, hormone regulation, and health maintenance. I even eat loads of bacon—fat and all! When I need an odd snack here or there, I choose something with protein and fatty, like a boiled egg, half an avocado, a tablespoon of coconut oil, nuts, or nut balls, or some leftover meat from the night before. If I want something a little sweet, I love to mash a couple tablespoons of coconut oil with some Medjool dates in a bowl for a sweet, gluttonous delight.

It is essential to consume a consistent daily supply of fat to fuel a healthy body. But don't let the simplicity of that statement mislead you. It is *not* an endorsement to eat *any* fat. Far from it. (I am not promoting deep-fried foods, biscuits, cakes, chocolates, etc.) The quality and source of fat is critically important. Eating the wrong fats causes inflammation in the body and is associated with nearly all lifestyle-related diseases: heart disease, type II diabetes, obesity, even cancer.

Provide your body the ingredients it is designed to use and trust that your body knows exactly what to do with them. Listen to the signals your body gives you, be present with its wants and needs, and your body will teach you. The way your abdomen and stomach feel day-to-day will teach you how correct you are with your food choices, and, as gross as it sounds, your bowel habit—that is the consistency, color, shape, and ease of your stools—also tells you how you are doing. I trust you know what I mean.

The way we viewed fats changed like never before in the 1950s, when the American academic Ancel Keys, PhD, proposed the theory that "proved" saturated fats caused heart disease and raised cholesterol levels. Although Keys changed his position over the next few years and made a number of inconsistent and contradictory statements, the damage was done and this led to widespread fear of saturated fats and cholesterol. By the 1960s, the promotion of the low-fat diet had begun, with deadly consequences to our health. This mistruth and avoidance of all fats, particularly saturated, built acceptance of highly processed and unnatural products like margarine and vegetable oils, and began the rise of trans fats in our food supply.

It has only been in recent years that a growing number of health authorities and scientists have realized trans fats are the real culprits in causing heart disease, and that specific types of saturated fats are actually highly beneficial. Unfortunately, despite having access to more and more updated information, many of today's doctors, nutritionists, and scientists and government bodies, cling tightly to the incomplete and faulty theories of half a century ago. This simply doesn't make sense to the logical mind, does it? Our government should want us to be healthy. Isn't health care costing billions, if not trillions, of dollars? Aren't we getting sicker and sicker? The reality is there is no time to lose waiting for others to care about our health, so let's be responsible for ourselves and our families and learn what *we* can do to stay healthy.

Fats are organic substances that are not soluble in water. *Saturated fats* are found in plant-based foods, such as coconut oil, cacao butter, palm kernel oil; and animal sources, such as milk, cream, cheese, butter, ghee, suet, tallow, lard, and meats. Choosing grass-fed meat is paramount because when it is from a bad source (i.e., conventional grain, hormone- and antibiotic-fed, stressed animals) it can be difficult for us to digest, not provide the needed nutrients, and heavy on our organs, such as the liver, kidneys, and pancreas. Good saturated fats are important for our brains, heart, liver, bones, lungs, thyroid, insulin levels, and many more vital body parts and functions.

Coconut oil has been shown to be the safest and most stable oil with which to cook.

Monounsaturated fats are found in natural foods, such as red meat, bacon, whole-milk products, almonds, pecans, cashews, peanuts, olives, and avocados. The oils from these are loaded with essential omega-3 fats, vitamins, and minerals. They are best eaten raw or slowly cooked. Drizzling olive oil over foods that are cooked is perfect, but not heating the oil to high temperatures, because unlike the other nut oils, olive oil is not stable under high heat. Monounsaturated fat is widely praised for reducing inflammation and lowering blood pressure.

Polyunsaturated fats include flax and flaxseed oil, chia seeds, primrose oil, borage seed oil, hemp and hemp seed oil, walnuts, leafy greens, fish, algae, and krill. Polyunsaturated oils are liquid, even when refrigerated, and are very unstable, going rancid easily. Polyunsaturated oils should never be heated or used in cooking. Omega-3 in particular must be treated with care. Unfortunately, Omega-3 deficiency is extremely common in wild game, and free-range meats and fish. Most diets are terribly low in this vital nutrient, and to make matters worse, many people over consume Omega-6 fatty acids, like those in corn and soy, upset the delicate balance between the two. This imbalance creates silent inflammation in the body, which leads to a myriad of chronic disease issues. Our over consumption of vegetable oils, combined with our consumption of processed grains, both of which are high in Omega-6 contributes to this imbalance. (This is why I take a quality fish oil supplement rich in Omega 3 every day, ensuring the fish used have been fished sustainably from clean waters and are low in mercury and other toxic pollutants.)

There are other fats that you should be aware of. In order to have unsaturated fats last longer and to make them look more appealing, food manufacturers use a process called *hydrogenation*. Hydrogenation takes unsaturated liquid fat (usually some kind of vegetable oil) and adds hydrogen, eliminating the double bonds in the carbon atoms. This makes the molecule more saturated. However, altering these fats makes them dangerous to consume, and they should be avoided. When unsaturated fats are only partially hydrogenated, a new type of fatty acid called trans fatty acids (TFAs) is created. These trans fats are destructive to the human body. They are found mostly in processed foods and commercial oils, and used to give cakes, pastries, and biscuits a more solid consistency, and to prolong shelf life. Trans fat is also found in vegetable shortenings, some margarines, crackers, and snack foods. It's an ingredient in the oils used to fry fast foods, like French fries and nuggets. *Choice* magazine found trans fats in meals sold at McDonald's and Hungry Jack's, in traditional meat pies, and even Nutella. Food labelling laws, unfortunately, are generally not on our side when it comes to trans fats. There are many loopholes to allow manufacturers to omit the words *trans fats* when it comes to labelling, even if the item does contain them. There are no tolerance levels in the body, although in Australia the "accepted" level is up to 2% trans-fat content for any given food. (In the U.S., it is mandatory to list the trans-fat content on packaging; in Australia, there is no such regulation.)

The good news is that food companies are gradually lowering the level of trans fats in their products as awareness of the dangers of them increase amongst consumers. This is particularly due to a series of court cases against large food companies like Kraft and McDonalds.

The consumption of trans fats promotes cell damage, premature aging, and increases the risk of coronary heart disease by raising levels of bad LDL cholesterol and lowering levels of good HDL cholesterol. Trans fats are so dangerous they have been banned in many countries.

According to the World Health Organization, avoiding TFAs is a must because TFAs damage the heart and have been linked to cancer, atherosclerosis, diabetes, obesity, immune-system dysfunction, birth defects, and problems with bones and tendons, Alzheimer's, liver dysfunction, and infertility in women. Simply put, do yourself a BIG favor and do not eat TFAs! Also, to be safe, avoid products with partially hydrogenated oil on their ingredient list and products high in fat that have a low saturated-fat content, as this often means the remainder is trans fats.

Deficiencies and omega fatty acid imbalance have also been shown to be a causal factor in developmental and behavioral issues with children. Signs of fatty acid imbalance, as stated in the book *Smart Fats* include dry skin, chicken skin on the back of your arms, dandruff, dry and unmanageable hair, soft and brittle nails, patches of pale skin on cheeks, cracked skin on heels or fingertips, lowered immunity, poor wound healing, frequent infection, dry eyes, frequent urination, fatigue, hyperactivity, learning problems, allergies, excessive thirst, etc.

Want more energy? One of the most outstanding benefits of consuming the right fats in the right ways (that is raw or heated, as discussed earlier) is the energy they produce. Coconut oil in particular, because it contains smaller fatty acids than most fats, is rapidly absorbed and used as immediate fuel for the body. This means quick nourishment is delivered without putting excessive strain on your digestive and enzyme systems. Missing out on enough fat is often one of the biggest contributors to the low-energy levels many people feel when trying to reduce weight or when starting a new diet, like Paleo, for example.

Good fats are also vital for efficient metabolism. A study in the *Journal of Nutrition* reported that researchers found that participants who consumed two tablespoons of coconut oil per day burned more kilojoules than those who consumed less. A speedy metabolism helps boost the body's digestive system and keeps weight off.

Eating enough good fat also stops sugar cravings. Instead of reaching for the candy to pick you up in the afternoon, when you would normally look for a sugar-hit, try eating some avocado or a small handful of nuts. Good quality fat is more satiating than carbs; so if you cut down on sugar, you will feel less ravenous. Constant hunger is often a major clue that your body is not being fed correctly. With proper amounts of fats and protein, you can fuel your energy reserves, and jump off the sugar roller coaster When you eat enough good fat, you'll feel more full and satisfied; and thus eat fewer calories overall.

You can be sure that if you come to my house for dinner, there will be fat! There will be nothing processed, no sugar, no grains, no trans fats, nothing out of a package, bottle, or wrapper, but loads of fresh wholesome foods from Nature. You will see me scoop tablespoons of coconut oil into the pan to slow cook the meat, and joyfully scoop one straight into my mouth at the same time. (Remember to open your mouth, because one will be coming your way too!) There will be salads with lots of different colored vegetables sprinkled with nuts, seeds, avocado, eggs, and olive oil. There will most likely be some raw (and fatty) cacao nut balls for dessert.

One way that I use fat, is for oil pulling. This is an ancient Ayurvedic practice to detoxify the body. It involves taking a tablespoon of oil (olive oil is fine, I use coconut oil which melts as soon as you put it in your warm mouth) into the mouth first thing in the morning, on an empty stomach, and swishing/rinsing it around, without swallowing, for approximately twenty minutes. Oil pulling draws out toxins and bacteria from between the teeth, and from gums and mouth tissues. These toxins often cause gum disease, tooth decay, and there is a now evidence of a connection between poor oral health and heart disease. The oil is then spat out and the teeth brushed and flossed, as per your normal routine.

As a caution, if you have been restricting fat in your diet for some time, increase the amount you eat slowly. When I started putting butter in my coffee, I had a tight and crampy stomach for nearly two weeks as my body adapted! The most common reported reaction to higher levels of fat consumption is diarrhea. An initial reaction of an unsettled stomach, breakouts of acne or flu-like symptoms are often a sign of the body detoxifying. Coconut oil in particular has anti-microbial properties that can cause a Herxheimer reaction, or die off, to occur as the body clears out unwanted pathogens (viruses, bacteria, fungus, parasites, etc.). This may pass after just a few days, and gradually increasing your fat intake is the key. Some people may mistake this reaction as a bad thing, but understand it is your body in all its wisdom using the new tools you are giving it to make necessary positive changes. Listen for these subtle cues and rest, nourish, and give your body time to heal.

When you make new decisions and take new action you do not only change your life, you change your family's life. I understand that things are often easier said than done, but I implore you to look beyond this and draw a new line in the sand. Take note, not only of what changes you would like to make, but why. What do you want to achieve and what is the driving force behind it? What does it mean about you? What is the emotion attached to the change? What's your real emotion deep down? Who are you doing it for? What are you teaching your children and the people in your life by demonstrating this behavior? How many more days of quiet desperation are you willing to have before making necessary changes? And, at what cost? Too often we make choices for the wrong reasons, or for someone else.

I understand firsthand that it can be soul-wrenching to watch someone you love on a self-destructive path, abusing their bodies with food or other substances. My father, whom I cherish and adore, has battled with his health and body for most of his life. He is on several medications; has had major surgeries; and suffers from heart disease, type II diabetes, and several neurological conditions. He is in constant agonizing pain, has lost feeling in his feet, is red-faced, exhausted, and short of breath. He does not exercise, does not drink water, does not eat living whole foods, and struggles with stress and sleep deprivation. Thank goodness he regularly receives Chiropractic care. If it wasn't for the benefits and hope that the Chiropractic philosophy imparts, he feels he would have given up long ago.

This is a constant source of heartache for me, as I see so much potential for my father's health and so much time lost feeling unwell, time lost that could have been spent enjoying life, enjoying his wife, children, and grandchildren. But, this is not my journey, it is his. It is my role to teach those who are open to learning better ways, and ready to take action. We can still love, accept, and respect those who choose another path, and use this as fuel and inspiration to treat our own bodies with more reverence.

You are on an extraordinary journey of discovery. Your level of wellness is increasing exponentially as you read this book. I applaud your evolution as it unfolds. Most people fail in life because they aim too low. Make sure you aim high and dream big. Please learn from my story and build the knowledge and confidence to listen to your Innate Intelligence. Your body is amazing. You are amazing. And you have an exceptional life ahead. There is nothing more beautiful than a person expressing his or her true, authentic self.

Enjoy your health, express curiosity and creativity, be strong, be more beautiful, enhance your leisure, relieve boredom, add fun to life, enjoy exotic tastes, and renew your vigor and energy. Live longer, learn, grow, and thrive!

Be bold and dream astronomically—and nothing will stop you!

About the Author

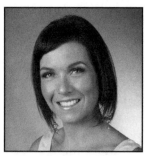

DR NATALIE BIRD is a chiropractor, author, speaker and health coach in Melbourne, Australia. She is dedicated to advancing public awareness about positive and proactive health care choices; and is often asked to write, blog, and speak for organizations with similar values. She is also a devoted wife, mother, and passionate lover of life.

Dr. Bird believes it is every person's universal and biological right to be strong, healthy, happy, and free. She teaches her patients that being healthy requires commitment, consistence, and an eager curiosity for knowledge. She knows how vital it is to have a support network of like-minded people, friends, and mentors who motivate and encourage you to continually advance and evolve your health choices and your lives. Her goal is to inspire others to be active participants in their own health care and well-being, and to be creators of their own health destiny through conscientious and empowered living.

Dr. Bird is a member of the Chiropractors' Association of Australia, the International Chiropractic Pediatric Association, and is a research partner of the Australian Spinal Research Foundation. In addition to five-year double bachelor degrees in Chiropractic Science and Clinical Science, she has completed thousands of hours of post-graduate training in Chiropractic technique, patient education protocols, and patient communication. Dr. Bird has extensively studied integrative nutrition as it relates to health and longevity, with a primary focus on grain and sugar-free Paleolithic eating.

Her patients include elite athletes, like Olympic medalists, AFL and A-League footballers, National champions in lacrosse, badminton, martial arts and athletics; employees of major corporations like Ford, Holden, and Telstra; as well as thousands of families.

For more information, please visit her website, www.platinumchiro.com.au.

To share your story, vision, or health epiphanies with Dr. Bird, you can also contact her at:

Platinum Chiropractic & Wellbeing
98A Douglas Parade
Williamstown, Victoria, AUST, 3016
Phone: +61 (03) 9399 9509
Email: drnat@bigpond.net.au
www.facebook.com/platinumchiro

"Regular Chiropractic care
saves lives, adds life to your years,
and years to your life."

GILLES A. LAMARCHE, DC

CHAPTER SEVEN

Your Plan Is Not Always God's Plan

Dr. Dustin Barton

The Art *of Being Healthy* is much more than the average self-help book as it contains secrets from like-minded humanitarians who live lives of abundant health. I have three clear objectives: the first is to challenge your current beliefs concerning health. Do you believe health comes from a bottle, potion, lotion, pill, or surgery? If you have symptoms, does that mean you are sick; and if you don't have symptoms, does that mean you are healthy?

The second objective is to identify the origin of human health. When you have a foundation on which to start, you are enabled to make congruent health choices.

Lastly, everyone has a story, aka a reason why they choose what they choose. Maybe something happened to make you believe health is based on genetics and, thus, you cannot make a difference in your future health.

People hear many statements that are, frankly, false. For example: If you have a headache, the solution is acetaminophen or ibuprofen. If you have heartburn, the answer is an antacid. As you get older, you will get arthritis. And, my personal favorite is: Chiropractic only helps neck and back pain.

I challenge you to identify the lies you have been told about health and the ones you believe. This is not to say you are wrong, but perhaps someone else's incorrect philosophy of health has had a major influence on your thinking.

One of my favorite quotes is: "If you don't think for yourself, someone will think for you." The truth of this statement is evident as you watch the constant blitz of commercials on TV (paid for by companies looking to make a profit) about what drug you need versus what health choice is best.

Do you believe that now or later is the time to make changes in your health paradigm? Here is a better question: will better health decisions today impact your health and that of your family tomorrow? Why wait to make better choices? Join me as I take you on a journey of life, a journey that has already served thousands by allowing them to better understand that they have the power to make better choices as it concerns their health and that of their family.

Please rewind to when you were a child. Were you aware of your purpose in life? I will always remember when I was twelve years old and my life was forever transformed by the power of the Chiropractic adjustment ...

Residents of Jamestown, North Dakota, recognize that hot summer days are quite limited. As a result, when a gorgeous, sunny day arrives, people flock to the local lakes to enjoy time with their friends and families.

It was a beautiful summer day in 1993, in Jamestown. I was twelve years old. The events of this day would lead me to my purpose for being on Earth. The sun was shining, as smiles and laughter filled the beach of a lake two miles outside of my hometown. On this day, I met another twelve-year-old boy who would be an inspiration to me for the rest of my life. I met him as people gathered on the west side of the lake to observe a friend parasailing.

If you're not familiar with the sport of parasailing, allow me to set the scene for you. Parasailing involves the use of a boat and a two- to three-inch thick towrope connected to the back end of the boat. In this case, it was an undersized speedboat. At the other end of the rope, approximately 150 feet away, is an individual connected to a parachute and holding onto the rope. The objective is to have the boat pull the individual some thirty to fifty feet in the air behind the boat. The experience of watching someone parasail is amazing.

Most of the thirty-five onlookers knew this was the man's first time parasailing. The ignition was turned on, and the loud motor of the speedboat echoed across the lake. The people in the boat yelled to the man, "Are you ready?" The man gave a two-thumbs-up signal and the driver of the boat hit the throttle.

Thud! Thud! That is the next sound I remember hearing. You see, there was a 20-30 mph breeze and the parasailing experience had been postponed three different times that day.

As the driver of the boat pushed down on the throttle, a gust of wind simultaneously came rushing through and spun the individual who was parasailing out of control. Thirty-three women, men, and children had their eyes on the parasail, but two children were focused on the fascinating sound screaming from the motor of the speedboat. As the individual parasailing tried to control his direction, the wind overpowered him. The result was two children were struck by the rope of the parasail.

The two thuds were the sound of the rope being strung tight and striking the chests of the two children. The rope struck child B square in the chest and carried him approximately ten feet before the rope slipped up over his chest, throat, chin, and off his face while slamming the boy's head off of a boat dock, leaving him unconscious.

The rope struck Boy A in the chest as well. Boy A was flung fifteen feet into the lake. As people rushed to Boy A's rescue, they were shocked to see that the pole of a dock was sticking out from his chest. However, by the grace of God, as they got closer, they realized that the pole was actually between his right arm and chest. The pole had glanced off his rib cage and missed puncturing his chest cavity by mere inches.

Months of healing from multiple skin lacerations were needed for both children. One terrible accident, on what can be viewed as one of my worst days, also became the most amazing day of my life.

> "What I do today is important because
> I am exchanging a day of my life for it."
> UNKNOWN

There comes a point in life when you might believe the world is completely against you. I vividly remember Boy B's life story. For the twelve years prior to this accident, this young boy had what many would consider normal health issues. Every year he was diagnosed with bronchitis and/or pneumonia. Week after week, year after year, more medications and higher doses were prescribed, yet his symptoms continued to get more severe.

Let's analyze the situation. Imagine the frustration for the family. Prescription drugs became the only answer to this child's health issues. Let me pose a question to you. If you were a doctor of medicine, how many times would you prescribe medications before you realized you didn't have the answer to this child's health issues? How long would it take? Five weeks? Seven months? Ten years? Is there a definite number?

Later in the summer of 1993, Boy B's health spun out of control. He was diagnosed with new health conditions, such as adolescent asthma, a concussion, and headaches. There were no specific reasons given as to why the asthma suddenly reared its ugly head. (Obviously, the blunt force of his head hitting the dock would explain the concussion and headaches.) The cause of his asthma was unknown. The boy and his family were told that he would need an inhaler for all sports, for the rest of his life, which was the common prognosis for asthma sufferers. Once again, another prescription drug was the answer.

The definition of *insanity*, as stated by Albert Einstein, is "Doing the same thing over and over and expecting a different result."

While sitting at the bottom of the stairs in his home, in August 1993, Boy B contemplated his life. As a twelve-year-old, he thought he had taken on more than he could handle in regard to his health. With a history of always being sick in the winter, constant headaches, a concussion that played havoc on his thinking processes and attitude, and being limited with asthma, where else was he to turn? Keeping to himself, he decided that this day was when all the issues would end. With a shotgun in his hand, he was prepared to do the unthinkable, especially for such a young boy. With no one else at home, his loneliness was all he had to hold onto.

BANG! The sound ended one life and another life began.

The sound of a door slamming shut and someone running into the house startled Boy B. It was his younger brother. For Boy B, his younger brother immediately became his hero and his best friend.

The life I have today started in August of 1993. I am Boy B. After years of being "doctored," it took a terrible accident with a parasail and another close call with death to find my True Health Potential as well as my Soul Purpose in Life! I cannot say enough about the true hero in my life—my brother!

> "God will not look you over for medals,
> degrees or diplomas, but for scars."
> ELBERT HUBBARD

God has a divine plan for us all and it is an individuals' series of choices that determine if he/she is living out their Soul Purpose. My brother saved my life and it was a Doctor of Chiropractic who would set me sailing free from the burdens of health issues and disease. I did not believe in Chiropractic, but I soon realized I did not have to believe in it for Chiropractic to work.

After a few months of receiving adjustments, my headaches, bronchitis/pneumonia, asthma, and depressive state disappeared. Had the medications finally worked? I vividly remember asking the Doctor of Chiropractic how he was able to find and correct my health issues. He said, "A Doctor of Chiropractic performs an adjustment to specific areas of the spine in order to improve the nerve communication from the brain to your muscles and organs. In other words, you cannot express 100% health if there is a disturbance in the nervous system (a subluxation)."

Chiropractic is a profession that abides by the natural laws of life.

Living a life of Soul Purpose is staying congruent with your personal philosophy of life in such a way that you never "work" a day in your life and leave all burdens aside.

"You cannot leave a place you have never been."
AYN RAND

Life provides us with many challenges, all of which are the proper stepping stones needed to achieve optimal health. As I described above, the only concept I was taught about health was that if you had symptoms you were to go to the medical doctor. In my experience, an MD typically has four options: to prescribe a drug, administer another vaccination, make a referral to another doctor in the hospital system, or suggest surgery.

Some quick questions: how many times must your heart beat per minute? What tells it to do so? How many breaths must your lungs take per day? How does your immune system respond to bacteria/viruses that surround you? What specific nutrients need to be synthesized in order to organize continued health?

I ask that you not worry about the answers to these questions, as the combined wisdom of the most brilliant scientists and doctors would never be capable of mastering such feats. The body has an inborn wisdom called *Innate Intelligence* that organizes all bodily functions. You are not responsible for organizing the function of your body, but you *are* responsible for the environment in which your Innate Intelligence must adapt.

No two humans are in need of the same physiological response at the same time, allowing for an individual to adapt to his environment easily or with difficulty. Have you ever been in a room or place of business where people are sick? Why do some get sick while others don't? Is it luck? If a bacteria and virus cause illness, wouldn't we all be sick at the same time? How do some people avoid illness? If genes were all that mattered, why don't all family members have the same disease/illness?

Your answers to these questions are soon to come!

Over the past twenty years, I have been blessed to meet many of the world's best philosophers, many of the greatest Doctors of Chiropractors, as well as other health professionals. They all agree on three foundational Principles of Life:

- The body is self-healing and self-regulating
- The nervous system is the Master System of the body
- Disturbance to the nervous system reduces one's expression of optimal health

Do you recall my health expression while experiencing nervous system disturbance (subluxation)? The Chiropractic adjustment was the answer. The goal of the above list and the remainder of this chapter are to challenge what you have been taught about health. Most of what you were taught was via your MFTP network (mother, father, teacher, preacher). Examples of what you may have heard about health are:

- Genes control health

- Health is luck

- Health issues and/or disease are hereditary and run in the family

I want you to have an open mind as you question some of your concepts about health because in order to live an extraordinary life, you must understand and/or question how you arrived at your current state. If anyone in your family has ever taken a medication for a cough, fever, sore throat, upset stomach, itchy eyes, allergies, asthma, runny nose, pneumonia, bronchitis and/or, but not limited to headaches, then the next half of this chapter is a must-read for you!

Your philosophy on health is the foundation on which you build your "temple" of health. Let's begin with a simple question. If you cut yourself, do you tell your body how to heal the cut? Of course not! Without applying a Band-Aid would your body heal the cut? Of course, it would. The human body is equipped with the most amazing health professional possible. The *Doctor Within* can never be outsmarted. *Innate Intelligence* is the specific name given to the Doctor Within.

Everyone has Innate Intelligence that continually constructs and organizes their physiology. The finite (educated) human mind could never, nor will it ever, be able to coordinate and organize the human body like Innate Intelligence is able to. Allow me to provide examples of the wisdom of Innate Intelligence. Innate Intelligence is found throughout your entire body, not one specific place. Innate Intelligence continually functions at 100%, continually adapting to the universal forces (stress) of life (physical, chemical, and emotional).

Doubting Innate Intelligence would be similar to doubting that the Earth is round or that gravity does not exist. Innate Intelligence is that perfection within all of us that formulated two cells (male sperm with the female egg) into an amazing human being nine months after conception. Throughout the entire pregnancy, the fetus's Innate Intelligence has guided growth, 24/7. Uniting the physical being with Innate Intelligence is the key to our existence.

Innate Intelligence is extremely efficient and always on the job.

These examples of the coordination and organization of Innate Intelligence are nothing short of amazing:

- The human heart beats approximately 100,800 times/day
- We take 18,000 to 30,000 breaths/day
- An individual blinks approximately 9,600 times/day
- A 150 lb. person has approximately ten to twelve gallons of water in his/her body
- The equivalent of 5,500 gallons of blood are pumped throughout the body daily
- The body contains approximately twenty-five feet of intestinal tract
- If put end to end, the nerves in your body would stretch around the entire Earth two and a half times

Every organ, cell, and tissue in your body is reliant on the other. Imagine your body as an orchestra. Innate Intelligence is the harmony (health) of all the instruments (organs) synchronized. Remove one or a couple of the instruments (organs) from the orchestra (body) and the harmony is still present, however one mistake could be noticed because there are less specific instruments (organs) contributing to the harmony (health). Innate Intelligence is the unseen, intangible conductor of the body that brings about the harmony of human life that you enjoy. The magic is not in the instruments (organs). The magic is in the coordination and organization which creates harmony (health). That magic is the conductor (Innate Intelligence).

Imagine if you removed a couple instruments (organs) from the orchestra. Not truly understanding the harmony (health) of an orchestra, you add something foreign to it, such as drums (medications) and guitars (vaccinations). Then, instead of grouping the same instruments (organs) together you spread similar instruments throughout the orchestra. The music will be played, but the harmony (health) is not optimal like it was before you intervened.

The human body is more complex than any instrument, machine, or living organism. In order for any organism to survive, it must adapt; and the human body has an amazing ability to adapt. Remember when your child first attempted to stand and walk? How well did that go? Did he/she ever fall? Because children at that age are too young to speak well, you relied on your power of observation to care for them. If your child was cut, you knew something traumatic happened, but if there was no evidence of trauma, you probably assumed all was well. At times, that might not necessarily be the correct assumption, right? (I know you are smart and answered yes.) Does the absence of symptoms or visible difficulty necessarily mean your child is healthy? When there is injury, does healing occur immediately? If you answered no to the last two questions, you are absolutely right.

One of life's principles is that all processes require time. For example, if you ever had braces on your teeth, you know it takes time to correct the alignment.

Let's revisit the example of a child growing from infancy to early childhood. Would it make sense that the 5,000 apparently minor falls may, in time, cause back pain, headaches, migraines, neck aches, knee issues, shoulder problems, etc.? If your answer is no, I ask you to fall an average of 5,000 times over the next five years and see how well your body functions. Remember, children aren't able to fully communicate how they feel with words until they are six or seven.

The definition of *health* is "the state of being free from illness or injury" (he was restored to health, "a health risk). The World Health Organization states: "Health is a state of complete physical, mental, and social well-being and not merely the absence of disease or infirmity."

Dissecting the World Health Organization's definition of *health*, it is clear to see that there are three factors that need to be complete: physical, chemical, and emotional stress. Physical stress encompasses but is not limited to the stress of sitting, standing, car accidents, falling down (bumps and bruises), exercising, driving in a vehicle, and sports. Chemical stress encompasses but is not limited to the stress of nonorganic foods, pesticides, herbicides, house-cleaning products, detergents, tap water that is "chemicalized," plastic glasses, vaccinations, medications (prescribed and nonprescription), air fresheners, perfumes, and/or environmental factors, etc. Emotional stress encompasses but is not limited to positive thoughts, negative thoughts, verbal abuse with spouse and/or children, job duties/deadlines, financial stress, and/or the balance of all emotions.

Life is filled with stressful events. Stress is considered to be universal and your Innate Intelligence has the primary responsibility to adapt to all of your life stressors. Many people believe they don't have stress in their life, are currently without symptoms, and thus healthy.

We all have stress. In fact, you are experiencing some form of stress right now. You are thinking (emotional stress), you are more than likely sitting (physical stress), perhaps you are straining your eyes from reading (stress), gravity is pulling on your body (physical stress), and you may have eaten processed food today (chemical stress). Consider your environment. What is in the air that you are breathing? Is your current posture detrimental to your health? Reading, most would agree, is a relatively low-stress activity, however stressors of all types are encountered daily. How do you believe your body performs during other activities and situations?

Hopefully you are now more aware of the stress that surrounds you and over time will have a greater ability to manage the stressors and overcome the possible negative effects of stress. Stress will never be something you can completely avoid, however you can optimize your body's ability to adapt to stress. ADAPTability is vital for survival. The human brain and nervous system are the most complex organisms known to man. Would you like to know how you can optimize your health by better adapting to the stress in your life? We all encounter similar chemical, emotional and physical stressors. Depending on the study, approximately 90% of all people now work at a desk. Our repetitive daily routines gradually inhibit the likelihood of experiencing our optimal potential as human beings.

Today, the majority of Americans wake up, skip breakfast, get their children dressed, go to work (where they sit or stand all day), do not eat a nutritious lunch, race to pick up their children from school or daycare, pick up fast food/pizza on their way home, watch television/play video games, go to sleep, and wake up to do it all over again! Days, weeks, months and years pass by and this lifestyle continually suppresses yours and your family's overall health.

How do you believe your current lifestyle will impact the health of your children? Let's look at more examples of lifestyle stressors in order to clarify the current lack of health in our communities. (The United States is one of the unhealthiest countries in the world.) Some additional examples of repetitive stress are:

• Eating fast food versus homemade meals

• Going to a job you dislike (coworkers, long days, duties)

• Do you work in a factory, sit at a desk and/or constantly do the same motions at work?

• Lack of valuable family interaction. How many hours a day to you positively interact with your children?

• Lack of exercise. Do you exercise regularly?

• Lack of "you time." Do you have leisure activities, hobbies, and/or other fun activities in order to relax?

"A wise man should consider that health is the greatest of all human blessings."
HIPPOCRATES

In order to experience a life of abundant health, you must focus on health rather than the *avoidance of disease*. Unfortunately, people have been brainwashed into thinking that good health is based on luck. In order to be diagnosed with a disease, one must lose health. To provide more clarity on the origin of health, let's identify the process of acquiring health.

The following quote from Dr. Lipton identifies how we constantly adapt to our environment, throughout all stages of life. The great news is that genes are no longer the focus for health. The focus of health stems from your lifestyle choices; so, choose wisely!

"Nature spends a lot of effort and energy in creating a child, and it doesn't do so randomly or just on a whim. Nature wants to ensure that a child is going to be successful in its life before embarking on the process of birthing that child. Although a child receives genes from both its mother and father, the genes are not fully set into the position of activation until the process of development. The first eight weeks of a child's development is called the embryo phase, and that's just a mechanical unfolding of genes to make sure the baby has a body with two arms, two legs, two eyes, etc. The next period of life is called the fetal stage, when the embryo has the human configuration. Since it's already shaped, the question is, what will Nature do to modify or adjust this human in the next number of months before it is born? What it does is this: Nature reads the environment and then adjusts the final tuning of the genetics of the child based on what's immediately going on in the world. How can nature read the environment and do this? The answer is that the mother and the father become nature's Head Start program. They're the ones who are living in and experiencing the environment. Their perceptions of the world are then transmitted to the child.

We used to think that only nutrition was provided by the mother to a developing child. The story was, genes control the development, and the mother just provides nutrition. We now know, of course, that there's more than just nutrition in blood. Blood contains information about emotions and regulatory hormones and the growth factors that control the mother's life in the world in which she's living. All this information passes into the placenta along with nutrition. If the mother is happy, the fetus is happy because the same chemistry of emotions that affect the mother's system are crossing into the fetus. If the mother is scared or stressed, the same stress hormones cross and adjust the fetus. What we're recognizing is that, through a concept called epigenetics, the environmental information is used to select and modify the genetic program of the fetus so it will conform to the environment in which it's going to grow, thus enhancing the survival of the child. If parents are totally unaware, this creates a great problem—they don't know that their attitudes and responses to their experiences are being passed on to their child."

The human brain has 100 billion neurons and stores more than 100 trillion bits of information. The brain is always in control and continually regenerates new cells, even in adults. If those numbers aren't staggering enough, your brain communicates via the spinal cord to every cell of your body through forty-five miles of nerves. It is said that human nerves relay over three million messages every second between the brain and every cell in our body at speeds up to 170 mph. The vitality of your life rests in a properly functioning nervous system. (If the media released this information about health on a daily basis, as much and as often as they do about disease and drugs, would there be a difference in the public's view of health?)

It is important to know that good health is not based on luck; it is, in fact, based on lifestyle choices. You are not experiencing headaches, irritable bowel syndrome, allergies, asthma, heart conditions, liver issues, and/or any other symptom because your body is lacking medications. Medications serve a purpose in that they dull the symptoms—but they are not a solution to health. If medications "help" a sick person become "well," then why wouldn't medications make someone who is well, "more well?" Health does not come in a plastic or glass bottle. What we do know is that your body has an infinite wisdom (Innate Intelligence) bottled up within every cell.

Your job is to continually seek a life that optimizes your health potential.

If life flows through the nervous system, what happens to your health if there is interference between the brain, nervous system (highway system connecting the brain to body), and body? People lose health anytime there is interference between the brain and body. If there is nerve interference, or what is more commonly referred to as *subluxation*, the expression of life is inhibited.

Approximately 8-12% of the nervous system is sensory. The remaining 88-92% of the nervous system does not relay pain/sensory signals. Would you board a plane that has a chance of making a safe landing only 8-12% of the time? Of course, you wouldn't. The question you must ask yourself is why are you living with the idea that if you don't have symptoms or feel pain you are healthy? Remember 88-92% of the nervous system controls functions of your body that you are unaware of on a second-to-second basis. What if there are communication issues within that 88-92% of your nervous system?

Would you allow your child in a vehicle with a drunk driver behind the wheel? This analogy is proposed because subluxations distort your body's expression of optimal health and reality, just as a drunk driver has a distorted view of reality. In other words, subluxations alter optimal health expression by inhibiting proper function of the nervous system. Subluxations are caused by physical, chemical, and emotional stressors. Your Innate Intelligence's primary function is to adapt to your lifestyle and environment (externally and internally). If Innate Intelligence is unable to fully express your health potential, your body begins to malfunction. A body that malfunctions enters a state of dis-ease and ultimately you encounter ill health. Medicine focuses on disease while Doctors of Chiropractic focus on the cause.. Subluxation is the cause of the dis-ease and ill-health, thus the logical solution to restoring health is to correct the subluxation.

The next time you or a family member experiences ill health, ask yourself why the body would respond in such a way. For example, is vomiting a good thing or bad thing? If your philosophy of health is that symptoms are bad, you may want to utilize drugs to suppress the vomiting. However, if someone is vomiting, isn't it true that the Innate Intelligence that controls and organizes all bodily functions is likely doing so to expel bacteria, viruses, and other pathogens that are harmful to your body? Do you truly want to suppress the symptom of vomiting?

What does a fever accomplish? Let's look at why we cook meat, such as chicken. One significant reason for cooking chicken is to kill off any bacteria or virus. If increasing temperature kills bacteria and viruses in the chicken, what do you believe takes place when Innate Intelligence creates increased temperature (fever) in your body? You are right. Increased body temperature occurs to help fight off infection.

Remember, health is a choice and you have the opportunity to start fresh on a daily basis. As a Doctor of Chiropractic, I am blessed to experience an abundance of health and I attribute my health to having a properly functioning nervous system, which in turn allows my Innate Intelligence to express health at 100%. Subluxation correction via the Chiropractic adjustment is, in my personal and professional opinion, the most valuable asset to human health.

If you want to experience an abundance of health, Chiropractic should be included in your lifestyle. I get checked for subluxations weekly. In fact, 90% of the practice members in my office have their entire family checked for subluxations one to four times a month.

If the following two questions resonate with your philosophy of health, make Chiropractic part of your lifestyle.

How well would you like your nervous system to function?

How long would you like your family's nervous system to function?

My hope is that your answer to these questions was a resounding 100%.

I envision a world in which all children achieve their optimal health potential.

My purpose is to inspire, enhance, and celebrate your family's life!

You can have all the riches in the world; however, without your health, you will never be able to enjoy the tangible and intangible assets the world has to offer!

About the Author

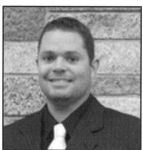

DR. DUSTIN BARTON obtained his Bachelor of Science in Marketing and Management from Minot State University in Bottineau, North Dakota, and the University of Minnesota, Crookston, in May 2003. Upon graduating from Northwestern College of Chiropractic in Bloomington, Minnesota, Dr. Barton interned at Nokomis Chiropractic in Minneapolis and Pfeffer Chiropractic in Alexandria, Minnesota.

In 2008, Core Health Chiro opened its doors on the principle foundation that the human body is self-healing and self-regulating. Dr. Barton is the founder, owner, and Doctor of Chiropractic within the business of Core Health Chiro. Dr. Barton and his team have a focused commitment to providing the highest quality Chiropractic care possible to the community. To maintain this commitment, they use the latest high-tech assessment equipment called the Insight Subluxation Station. The Insight Subluxation Station is a scanning technology that enables patients to better understand the benefits of regular Chiropractic care in achieving overall wellness.

His life purpose is to help people of all ages heal naturally (without medication or surgery), through the principled, scientific approach of subluxation and wellness-based Chiropractic.

Dr. Barton was recognized and awarded Chiropractor of the Month for May 2012, by On Purpose, a premier organization that recognizes excellence and a chiropractor's commitment to the public and to the Chiropractic profession by advancing wellness.

In recognition of his achievement, Dr. Barton was interviewed and featured on On PurposeTM, the monthly audio subscription service produced by On Purpose, LLC, where he discussed his involvement in: Community Health Outreach Programs (available to organizations, churches and/or business), EPOC (an organization established to enhance the Chiropractic profession), as well as maternal and infant health. Dr. Barton also discussed his love for serving and involvement as it relates to BNI and the Fargo Kiwanis organizations.

In May 2013, Dr. Barton was interviewed on the "Wellness Matters" radio show, based in St. Louis, Missouri. The live interview was centered on the topic of maternal and pediatric health and reached 200,000 plus listeners.

In 2013, Dr. Barton began traveling the U.S. speaking to businessmen and women, as well as organizations within the Chiropractic profession. Dr. Barton has chosen to expand beyond his community in order to continue fulfilling his Soul Purpose. Plans of traveling the world speaking on topics related to Chiropractic and health will soon come to fruition.

To make a health appointment for you and your family, or to book Dr. Barton as a guest speaker for your workplace, church, or civic organization, please visit his website: www.corehealthchiro.com.

You can also contact Dr. Dustin J. Barton at:

Core Health Chiro
4955 17th Avenue S., Ste. 108
Fargo, ND 58103
Phone: (701) 364-2673
Email: drbarton@corehealthchiro.com
www.facebook.com/corehealthchiro

*"While other professions are concerned
with changing the environment
to suit the weakened body,
Chiropractic is concerned with
strengthening the body
to suit the environment."*

B. J. Palmer, DC

CHAPTER EIGHT

Health Is a Journey, Not a Destination

Dr. Bettina Tornatora

I looked at the woman standing in front of me. Her eyes were wet with tears. "Oh my goodness, I feel like I am seeing him properly for the first time," she said.

I handed her son to her and she held him close; the connection was palpable. I knew I had just witnessed another Chiropractic miracle.

At six weeks of age, this baby was unhappy. He had cried all of his life, and had very little time of peace. His face was perpetually red and completely contorted into a painful grimace. He fed often but was rarely satisfied, and fussed so much at his mother's breast, that he had split her skin many times. His mother was exhausted as she had not been able to put him down for more than minutes at a time since his birth.

As I removed the pressure in his upper neck, the effect was spectacular. He relaxed his whole body and his face took on a beautiful, cherub-like expression. It was this child I handed back.

Later that same day, I was in our reception room. I saw a wonderful client who was in her late eighties. She was unable to drive to our office from her retirement village, and had arrived early for her adjustment, as taxi rides had proven unreliable in timing. After years of coming to be adjusted in the morning, her appointments had changed to the afternoon. As I greeted her, she shared the reason for this change.

At her new retirement village, as a matter of policy, she was now under the care of the General Medical practitioner for the village. This MD visited the village daily in the mornings, to attend to any residents who were in need. He had noted the woman's absence some mornings and asked her where she went. She shared that she visited the chiropractor. He reacted negatively to this revelation and told her Chiropractic was dangerous to her health at her age. Subsequently, the MD created pressure for her not to attend.

"So, I told him I would consider it," she said. "I mean, he did not want to hear that it was important to me, or that I have been doing this for nearly fifty years. It is what keeps me going. Then, I called the office and asked them to move my appointments to the afternoons from now on."

I must have looked perplexed as to how this changed anything.

"Well," she said, "he leaves at lunchtime and what he does not know won't hurt him. I am going to choose what is good for my body!"

These stories are not rare. In fact, most chiropractors have similar stories. What struck me on this particular day was the contrast in ages of these two clients and the way they represented the continuum of health. The beginning of life and the end stages are unique, as is every stage along the way. Our health is truly a journey, with many twists, turns, joys, and challenges. To achieve health is temporary harmony and this is the completely natural and normal human nature of the body.

Achieving a sense of harmony is a goal worth striving for. As you paint the picture of your health, you are the artist who keeps producing, and it is important to understand that this is a process. Chiropractic is a vehicle that allows your body to achieve its best harmony. No matter where you begin, no matter your age, or your circumstance, when you allow the body to fully express itself through a magnificent nervous system, a masterpiece is created.

Balance or Harmony?

The definition of *balance* is equal and opposing elements that reach equilibrium. The picture we often envision is of scales and balance beams. This view indicates that challenges will upset the balance and create disruption to the system. The maintaining of a system that is finely and possibly precariously balanced is very energy-consuming. There are many vital systems in our bodies that require a different method. In fact, they rely on a system of challenge and difference rather than a balance to function well. Some examples are:

Our vital **cardiovascular system** relies on variances of pressure, both throughout the blood vessels and internally in the heart to maintain a rhythmic harmony. The cardiovascular system is a closed system which means that the blood circulates within it and it exerts a force on the blood. Because liquids cannot be compressed, this force creates a pressure. There are two key factors here. Firstly, the existence of pressure in the various components: the heart, arteries, capillaries, and veins; and secondly, the *difference* in pressure between these components. If the pressures remained the same, the equality would create stagnation, or no movement. In fact, the gradient or difference between the pressure exerted by the blood and the resistance in the vessels of the system are what create the flow for the circulation to occur.

In this system, the body is certainly never striving for balance but rather a harmony utilizing differences and challenge.

The **nervous system** is made up of cells that transmit impulses throughout the body. The impulses have a domino effect of transferring from one to the other via an amazing system of movement of substances in and out of the cells. This movement is reliant on the charge or ions in and out of the cell membranes. What is significant about this system is that when the nerve is effectively resting, there is a total balance of charges between the inside and the outside. In a way, this is a resting state and messages are not being transmitted. When the impulses travel along the nerve to create some effect in the body, there is movement of the ions, or in other words the charge and the *difference* creates the nerve to move the impulse, moving the message from nerve cell to nerve cell. The alterations of specific chemicals create the action to occur.

These systems are not trying to achieve an equal and opposite balance; rather a harmony of the elements to achieve an outcome that is favorable. In addition, these systems are able to adapt and change to our circumstances. When we are under physical load and exerting ourselves, our bodies change our heart rate, blood pressure, and pulse to accommodate this. We are then better able to perform the task at hand. In fact, the problems begin to occur when our bodies are unable to make the changes to accommodate our exertions.

To take this one step further, we are able teach our bodies to allow the fluctuations to be minimal and the effect improved. This is seen in the case of physical exercise. When we do an activity regularly over time our bodies learn to change more quickly and recover more rapidly. In this way, we create a new and improved set point in our internal environment. When we first learn a movement, we are challenged; and as we adapt, our nervous systems work faster and more efficiently to enable us to perform it better and better.

Much of this change and challenge goes completely unnoticed by us. We do not know exactly when our blood supply to our muscles improves or our heart is stronger and able to pump more blood efficiently. We do not feel the changes in the firing of our nerve cells with our learnt movements and functions. Equally important, we do not know when it does *not* occur either.

This delicate harmony is maintained, controlled, and influenced by one sophisticated messenger system in the body—the nervous system. This is the central and governing control center for all the functions that occur. From the basic chemical changes to the largest movements there is nervous-system contribution.

What happens in the body when this harmony is interrupted? At first, we notice little change because our nervous system is calibrated to give few of its billions of messages as conscious pain or symptoms. In fact, by the time we know there is an interruption or interference happening in the body, there has been a significant change. By the time your body tells you that your systems are not working at their optimum, the harmony of your health has been compromised.

How Chiropractic Fits In

The chiropractor detects *subluxations*—regions of irritation to nerves in the spine. By removing these interferences, the chiropractor is allowing the body to strive for the harmony it naturally wants to achieve. When the central controlling system, the nervous system, improves in function, the entire body is affected. Over time, this allows the systems within to calibrate and create new set points.

Because the body is self-regulating and self-healing, this input can be significant to a person's health and allow the creation of a new way of being. The Chiropractic lifestyle involves regular removal of these subluxations via an adjustment and support for a person to understand how their bodies work.

When is the Ideal Time?

When I'm less busy. When I can afford it. When the kids go back to school. When I lose some weight. When the weather is warmer. When the weather is cooler. When I turn thirty, forty or fifty. When exams are over. When I get promoted. When my wife has the baby. ... and on and on the reasons go. These statements are often heard when decisions need to be made to improve one's health.

The reason these statements seem valid by those who make them, is that they see this journey of health as a destination; a location that we arrive at to stake our flag into the earth and claim, "I'm healthy now!" It is the pounds lost, the fitness gained, the motivation accessed, and the goal achieved. It is the point where a person relaxes and enjoys the fruits of their labor and puff out their chest and say, 'I did it!' It is also often the place where the effort stops and the attention can be removed. When we see health this way, these reasons become valid, but what is on the other side of this triumph, is a return back to the way things were. As soon as you remove the attention to the goal of "getting healthy," all the benefits slowly disappear; so, excuses are made before they begin and avoidance is chosen.

This reasoning only makes sense if you see achieving health as a finite location to arrive at and not a continuous journey to enjoy.

At all ages and stages, our body is adapting and changing. The achievement of health is a journey that requires effort and energy along the way. There is no point where we say, "Now we don't have to think about this anymore." As we move through our lives, we encounter physical, chemical, and emotional/mental stressors and we make adaptations. Life is a challenge, in particular in this modern world of ours. Negotiating the bombardment of toxins and stressors that can come literally twenty-four hours a day for many years, challenges one's health. And these stressors are not exclusive to adults. Children younger and younger are demonstrating signs of stressful adaptation to their environments. Removing the effects of this on the body via the Chiropractic lifestyle is paramount to living an optimized healthy journey at any and all stages of life.

From one day to one hundred days old, up to 100 years of age, all are perfect beginning points to start your Chiropractic health journey. Of course, the earlier you begin to positively influence your health, the better. Prevention is always the preferred option.

However, you can begin the Chiropractic journey at any age. During my twenty years in practice, I have had clients of each and every age from newborns to ninety-eight years young; all different and ALL on a journey of their own. Unique and individual. What these people have in common is interference to their nervous systems that required correction, and the willingness to learn information about a better way to live and achieve better health.

Since you are reading this book, I assume that you realize there is no good time to allow the interference and the subsequent decrease in your health potential to be present.

Having this interference left undetected and uncorrected is of no benefit to you, and as a chiropractor I can help you, by determining the best course of care for you and create the optimum healing schedule for you to achieve optimum health.

What are Your Health Expectations?

We are all conditioned by our beliefs, and our beliefs about our health are powerful in creating our physical, mental, and spiritual condition. This phenomenon is discussed in great depth by many authors, including, Bernie Segal, Deepak Chopra, Wayne Dyer, Louise Hay, and Stephanie Dowrick, who speak of the power of a person's belief system and expectations on their health and their ability to heal.

How are these expectations formed? They arise from the learned conditioning that life has brought to you. The sum total of the experiences you have had. Your expectations can be anywhere along the spectrum from: total trust of your body and its ability to cure all or a complete loss of trust that the body is self-healing. These expectations can dictate your choices for your personal health masterpiece. These ideas are the framework you use to make decisions.

We can eavesdrop on what a person's expectations are. They may make statements like "My mother had that, so I will have that." "All the women in my family have that." "The men in my family all die early." "No one in my family has ever ..." This thinking creates change in the body that poisons your health. The mind is a powerful tool and people's thoughts create their reality.

A benefit to attending Creating Health Workshops in Chiropractic is that you might begin to question the ideas and concepts that you have held about your health potential.

A Chiropractic Assistant who joined our practice began to receive Chiropractic care regularly. (All team members are put on a schedule of Chiropractic care.) When beginning her schedule, she was in her late fifties and had never done any exercise other than the incidental movement gained by working or home duties. "I don't really like to sweat," she said when asked about exercise.

As her body began to respond to having its nervous system working optimally, she noted changes in many areas of her life. Her energy increased, her concentration improved, her tolerance to change increased, her weight decreased, her appetite changed, her immune system was stronger and fought infections better, she noticed that she took less prescribed medication, her skin cleared, and her eyes shone as they had when she was younger. Another fantastic change took place. She began to question her health expectations. She had previously attributed so many of the aspects of her poor health to her age or genetic makeup, and now everything was getting better. She began to understand that if age and genetic makeup had little to do with her previously poor health, what else needed to be questioned?

With Chiropractic care for the detection and correction of subluxations at the center of her new health care paradigm, she also began to exercise, walking daily at first, then joined a women's-only gym, then joined challenges in the gym. After ten years and now in her mid-sixties she trains every day, sweats regularly, and has competed in short-course running events. She has smashed through the restrictions of what she expected of her health and is living a much happier, healthier existence as a result.

This is a living example that it does not matter when you begin the journey. You and only you set the pathway, so long as you are prepared to ask the question "What really is possible for me?"

Another subject that this example demonstrates is taking action. Many people see their health as a passive exercise. They caught the cold their husband brought home from the office. Or they were struck down by the flu. Or their back just went out with no reason at all. These statements suggest that a person is at the mercy of whatever the world, or their body, throws at them—helpless and out of control.

With greater understanding of how the body functions, the concept that health is ultimately each individual's responsibility becomes the cornerstone of what is possible. In this way, the events around your health are seen as feedback for your actions and efforts.

Catching the cold that the husband "brought home" is likely a sign that both her and her husband have been stressed due to a family matter and therefore immune compromised. Maybe both have been worried about his mother, not sleeping well and depleting their energy and immunity, allowing bacteria to invade their bodies and create cold symptoms.

Or the "flu" that struck them down was on the Tuesday after the big family wedding where they had partied for three days straight, eating and drinking out of character for their normal ways.

Their back "going out" may have been related to extra work that they were taking home every night this month, working on the laptop, increasing their screen time, and sitting double the usual amount, with little or no breaks.

By thinking in a new, responsible way, the feeling of being victimized by your health is removed. It is replaced by a feeling that action can be taken to make you well and stay that way. Understanding that there is always something you can do to support your body—no matter what it is presenting to you—is powerful beyond measure. It begins the healing process and allows you to feel empowered by your choices.

Who Needs to Know This?

If you are reading this book, there is a chance you and your family already enjoy the benefits of Chiropractic. Or perhaps someone who loves you wanted you to read this because they have experienced this joy and wanted to share it with you. Either way, now that you have a greater understanding I ask you: "Who else needs to understand this information?"

Chiropractic has been around for over 118 years. It has been attacked and ridiculed and put under enormous pressure to change its views. What was previously considered Chiropractic theory and philosophy has gradually become science as we discover more and more about how the body works and thrives. Still, there are too few people gaining from this great gift and fully expressing their full potential. There is no sadder statement in practice than "I wish I had known about Chiropractic sooner." It breaks my heart to hear these words, yet I am always honored when someone chooses me as their family chiropractor, no matter where they are on their health journey.

"I wish I had known about Chiropractic sooner" really means "I understand I have lost time on my health journey" or "I could have had so much more."

Though I am saddened when I hear those words, this strengthens my resolve to share the Chiropractic story with as many people as possible. It makes me more determined than ever that every person who comes into my sphere of influence would have the opportunity to learn what I know. I take that responsibly seriously, and I ask you to share the message of hope with those you know and love. Will you express your full potential through Chiropractic? Will you share the power of the nervous system with all your loved ones and all the people you know?

I understand that this takes courage, and I appreciate it may be new to you to live this way. But what if you knew what I know, and that is, that you can change lives by sharing this information? Would you share lifesaving health information if you had it? Well, now you do—what are you waiting for? Together we can build a healthier planet.

~ ~

The little boy who showed himself completely to his mother in my office continues to improve. He feeds well. His two-year-old brother is happy to have some time with Mum again. He can sleep for hours without waking. And he smiles all the time. The rest of the family is amazed by the change, and this little man now has a clear canvas to create his health journey.

Our older female client with the reluctant MD continues to attend our office in the afternoons. She says she will have her Chiropractic lifestyle for as long as she lives. She is grateful to her neighbor who put her onto Chiropractic all those years ago and gave her the gift of this knowledge, and for all she has gained in the process. She looks back on her journey and sees it as a masterpiece of her creation, and sees it as "warts and all, but definitely unique."

Every day I awaken feeling blessed to be a chiropractor, and I am so very grateful to have the opportunity to share this truth with you.

About the Author

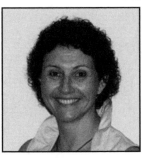

DR. BETTINA TORNATORA is a passionate person. She shares this passion through Chiropractic, writing, presenting, coaching, and living her purpose of love and service. She has practiced as a chiropractor for twenty years and, in this time, her focus has been on educating her clients on health, well-being, and making empowered choices.

Dr. Bettina and her husband, Jim, who is also a chiropractor, have been associate chiropractors, run rural practices, and satellite practices in very remote areas. They have worked with people of all ages and interests. In recent years, they have a family focused practice in inner western Melbourne. They have also become coaches and mentors for their profession.

A great focus of Dr. Bettina's work is the empowering of people to make great health choices. She is patient and understanding of the need to repeat this message until it is heard, no matter the situation. She believes that life is all about the journey, and that we must remain optimistic that it is never too late to learn or improve your life and health.

She is a loving mother of two amazing sons. She accredits much of her passion and inspiration to all her loving relationships. She believes that learning and growing on life's journey is truly a gift to be grateful for.

To schedule an appointment for you and your family, or to book Dr. Tornatora to speak at your workplace, church or civic club, please visit her website: www. bettinatornatora.com.

You may also contact Dr. Tornatora at:

Moreland Chiropractic
346 Moreland Road
Brunswick West
Melbourne Victoria Australia 3055
Phone: +61 3 9386 8451
Email: bettina@powerful-practices.com

CHAPTER NINE
Nutritional Balancing

Dr. Todd Lizon

In almost every Chiropractic office is a poster or brochure on physical, emotional, and chemical stress. There is a good reason for this: virtually every chronic degenerative problem has its origin in these factors. If you scratch the surface a bit deeper, there is another intriguing common thread in Chiropractic offices, and that is one of a holistic health paradigm. Chiropractors know that the body will heal on its own when any interference present is removed, and that treating the symptoms alone will not create health. To be healthy and vital, our physical, emotional, and chemical stresses must be addressed in a holistic paradigm. There is simply no other way.

With this holistic approach, how do most people actually deal with illness? If we honestly reflect on how the majority of the population deals with their health, some disturbing facts emerge. The reality is that most people go to their medical doctor, explain their symptom, and the vast majority of the time walk out with a prescription that will at best address the symptom but do nothing to address the root cause of the problem.

Fortunately times are changing. A growing percentage of the population is starting to understand that the present medical model is doomed to failure and that we must be addressing the root physical, emotional, and chemical causes of our health problems in a holistic paradigm of care. A large part of this holistic paradigm involves Nutritional Balancing.

Let's put this into a real life example. Take depression, diabetes, cholesterol, or thyroid issues. What do we do and whom do we see? Medical doctors are not going to have the answers unless they have a holistic approach and are willing to help patients address the root causes. While the intention of medical doctors is good, most unfortunately do not have the time or the knowledge of the holistic approach, and their tool bag is essentially limited to prescription medications that focus primarily on the masking or management of symptoms.

What about naturopaths? Well, unless they subscribe to the holistic paradigm of health and address the causes, this option is usually not much better. Using depression as an example, most naturopaths would prescribe St. John's Wort. While this may make the symptoms of depression better, it is fundamentally no different than the medications a medical doctor would prescribe in the sense that it is not addressing the cause.

What is one to do? If you want to be healthy, you need to seek out professionals who truly understand the holistic paradigm and address root causes. The holistic paradigm of always treating the cause is critical and is the central pillar of Nutritional Balancing. Nutritional Balancing is a program designed to bring the body into dynamic equilibrium and is an advanced method of healing that helps restore the body's vitality and energy-producing capacity by gently, but powerfully, balancing body chemistry rather than through the use of multiple remedies.

Understanding "The Change"

Nutritional Balancing is all about helping you get your health back; and I will outline in simple steps exactly how to do this.

Our starting point is the question that is asked in thousands of offices around the world every single day: How did I end up like this?

Intuitively, we know we didn't get sick in just one day, but most of us don't understand how we got sick. Here are the facts that will allow you to answer this most important question.

FACT #1: Physical, emotional, and chemical stresses are the negative driving factors of chronic degenerative disease.

FACT #2: If you can measure or see a change in your body, then your chemistry has changed from normal to abnormal.

The next critical question to ask, if you are to reclaim your health is: How did these stresses change my body chemistry from normal to abnormal?

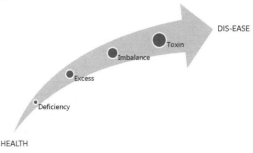

There are five factors that drive this process: genetics, deficiencies, excesses, imbalances, and toxins. If you wish to regain your health and reverse the dis-ease process, these factors must be dealt with in addition to the emotional, chemical, and physical stresses.

Let's briefly explore these driving forces because when you truly understand them, you will know more than many health professionals.

1. Genetics

In his book *The Biology of Belief*, Bruce Lipton sums it up beautifully. He writes that unless you are unfortunate enough to have a genetic disease expressed at birth, such as cystic fibrosis, then genetics is not what is causing you to be unwell. Genes need to be "turned on" or expressed if they are going to have an effect on the body.

The relatively recent discovery of epigenetics has shown that it is our environment that turns on genes. By environment we mean the physical, emotional, and chemical stresses we experience. If you have a gene for a particular condition, unless you trigger it with environmental factors, it will never express itself and the dis-ease will not develop.

The conclusion is that if you live a good, healthy, and clean lifestyle, your negative genes should never turn on and be expressed. Genes are not a significant factor in chronic degenerative disease and probably only apply to about 5% of the population. This is great news as it means the problem is lifestyle-based and can be addressed and corrected.

2. Deficiency

This is so simple and important; yet commonly overlooked. Here is the rule that you must always remember: all cells require nutrients to function. If the nutrient is not present, the cell will not function at its best. A simple example is oxygen. Without it, we have no life. Without our minerals and vitamins, we would face similar fates. With today's lifestyles and diets, it is not surprising that deficiencies are commonplace.

3. Excess

In our consumer-driven society, we are often led to believe that more is better. We buy into this in many subtle ways. One way is by using multivitamins indiscriminately. We tend to buy them as insurance policies and think that if we just keep putting more in, it will be good for us. This logic couldn't be further from the truth! Let's take Vitamin C as an example because, as it turns out, Linus Pauling had it wrong. He thought there was no way to have too much vitamin C, but the reality is that just as deficiency is an issue, excess is as well. If you have too little vitamin C, you will be immuno-depressed; if you have too much, you will become immunosuppressed. Either way, you experience a similar outcome. Supplements should be a critical part of your overall health plan, but you need to ensure that you are taking the right ones, in the right amounts, and on an individual basis.

4. Imbalance

Simply put, this is about getting the balance of your chemistry correct. The minerals in your body, for example, are in relationship with each other in a similar way that you are in relationships with your family and friends. Whatever you do, you need to take into account the effect it may have on your body. When you raise the level of a single nutrient, such as magnesium, you will affect the levels of at least two other minerals. (I'll explore this in more detail shortly.)

5. Toxins

Toxins have a far greater influence on your body than most people think—and everyone must deal with this growing problem. Toxins have the adverse effect of substituting or replacing the preferred nutrients in the body and they have the devastating effect of blocking the ability of the body to use nutrients, EVEN IF the nutrient is already present.

These five factors explain what the stressors are doing to you and are the missing link to being able to reverse the disease process. They are absolutely critical when we are looking to balance the body and slowly but surely restore a person's health. And all must be addressed when we are dealing with serious health challenges. A Nutritional Balancing program is designed to do this.

Nutritional Balancing: Reversing the Change

Nutritional Balancing takes a holistic approach to health and addresses your pathological lifestyle stresses and choices. When you remove the physical, emotional, and chemical stresses from your life, you can allow the natural, Innate ability of the body to heal itself.

In real life though, it is not always that simple. There are some stresses that you simply can't ignore, fix, or walk away from. Challenging children don't deserve to be abandoned. Financial trouble can't be ignored. In this scenario, you need to support the body in supplementary ways while putting plans in place to resolve the stresses over the longer term.

A Nutritional Balancing program works in two parts.

1. **Reduce or eliminate** your physical, emotional, and chemical stresses.

2. **Contain the stresses** you can't eliminate with diet, lifestyle, emotional growth, detoxification, Chiropractic, and correct supplements.

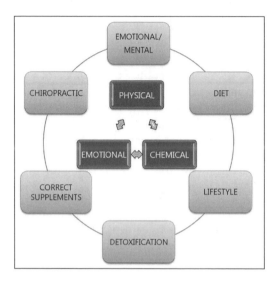

The diagram above illustrates the stresses (physical, emotional, and chemical) that are at the core of our health challenges; we must eliminate them when possible. The outer ring represents the ongoing battle to minimize our ongoing stress. The goal of the outer ring is to "contain" the stress and minimize its damage.

In a true holistic fashion, no one part is more important than any other, and they must all be addressed. In addition to Chiropractic, diet, lifestyle, and emotional well-being, Nutritional Balancing uniquely looks at detoxification and the use of specific supplements that are unique to an individual's needs. When assessed in a holistic way, this information on toxicity and correct supplements is not as well known or understood; and will, therefore, be the focus for the remainder of the chapter.

Hair Tissue Mineral Analysis—The Starting Point

Now that we have established that deficiencies, excesses, imbalances, and toxins are what drives our body chemistry from normal to abnormal, we need to focus on how to reverse the process. In order to do so, we need to assess and measure what is happening in the body. An individual's adaptation to stress will be unique; and so, we need to know where they are in order to start peeling back these "layers of adaptation."

The use of the right test is imperative. You would never use a blood test to assess a broken leg; the same logic applies to mineral, stress, and toxic-metal status. Chronic degenerative diseases occur in tissues, not blood; as a result, we need to assess what is happening in the tissues not only the blood.

A hair mineral analysis is one of the best ways to do this. As explained by Dr. Lawrence Wilson in his book Nutritional Balancing and Hair Mineral Analysis, the following are some of the reasons why hair is so valuable and informative.

1. The hair is a cellular biopsy. This means it provides information from the deepest level of metabolism, where most problems begin. For this reason, it often reveals imbalances long before symptoms or signs arise in the blood or elsewhere.

2. The body deposits toxic metals in tissues such as the hair to get rid of them. This can go on for years, until the body can no longer keep up this adaptive behavior. Only then does the problem cause symptoms or imbalances that are revealed on a blood test, for example.

3. The blood is generally maintained at the expense of tissues such as hair. For example, this means that a zinc deficiency will show up far sooner in the hair because the body will literally reroute zinc from the less important tissues to maintain the level in the blood and other vital organs.

A good way to think of a hair mineral analysis is as a screening test that measures the levels of minerals and toxic metals present in a sample of hair. Providing a "window into the cells," hair makes an excellent biopsy material and reveals a clear record of mineral metabolism.

Another significant benefit to Hair Tissue Mineral Analysis is that it reflects long-term metabolic activity as it measures an average of mineral accumulation over a three-month period. This is often an advantage, as the test results are not influenced by day-to-day variations in body chemistry due to stress, diet, or other factors.

Hair tissue is like a blueprint of one's individual biochemistry, and it can assist in identifying mineral patterns which may be associated with stress, blood sugar, and carbohydrate imbalances; metabolic rate; biochemical energy production; glandular imbalances; and more. It is also well established worldwide as a means to measure environmental contamination with toxic metals in the soil, plants, and human and animal populations.

Following is a hair mineral analysis chart to help you better understand why this is such an important tool in guiding the process of health restoration.

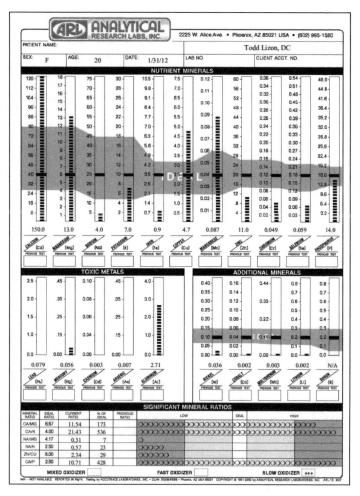

At the top of the graph is a section titled NUTRIENT MINERALS. Much like a blood test, there are established levels and these are visualized as the shaded area. Anything above or below the norm needs to be assessed and interpreted.

Below this is a section assessing TOXIC METALS. Of course, you don't want to see any toxicity in your hair analysis.

At the bottom of the page is a section called SIGNIFICANT MINERAL RATIOS which looks at some of the more important mineral relationships in the body.

It is important with a Hair Tissue Mineral Analysis to ensure that you understand what it is saying and what it is not. The basic rule to remember is that this test shows what is coming into the body, or what is leaving the body, during the three-month period that the hair was growing; nothing more and nothing less. Proper interpretation, much like an MRI or ultrasound, is critical.

What is This Hair Analysis Telling Us?

1. Deficiency. There are low levels of minerals such as iron, zinc, and selenium.

2. Excess. There are very high levels of calcium, copper, and manganese.

3. Imbalance. There are significant imbalances with Calcium to Magnesium (Ca/Mg ratio) and Sodium to Potassium (Na/K ratio)

4. Toxins. Mercury and aluminium are present.

Interpretation is critical.

When looking at the level of mercury in the example, you will see it is at 0.056 mg%. This tells us mercury is present, but it doesn't clarify if it was ingested or if the body was eliminating it. This is where the detective work (interpretation) comes into play. In our example, the person is young, has no mercury amalgams in her teeth, and eats a lot of tuna. When you consider her history, you can surmise that her high level would likely be from the mercury present in the tuna, which is not unusual.

Let's assume she cuts out all seafood from her diet and six months later retests. If the mercury shows up at the same level, then it can't be from the tuna. At this point, the conclusion would be she either has another source of ongoing exposure, or it is her body slowly and steadily eliminating it through her hair.

When we look at the results, we must always be aware that they are not showing total body load, only what is present in the hair during the period of time it was growing. Many people who use these tests would look at these results and say something along the lines of "her zinc is very low at 11 mg%; let's give her zinc." This is potentially dangerous and reckless; and is reductionist not holistic.

We need to stop and ask why the zinc is low in this person. In addition to a pure zinc deficiency, there are two main reasons zinc could be low on a hair analysis and they are critical to understand. Conceptually the reasons can be grouped into the categories of the "mineral wheel" and "toxic metals."

The Mineral Wheel

The law of cause and effect is one that most people are familiar with and it has massive implications for your health. One application of this law for optimal health is that of the mineral wheel.

It turns out that each mineral in our body affects the levels of all the other minerals in extremely specific and sometimes surprising ways. They are in a relationship, as are vitamins. Let's look at the following illustration.

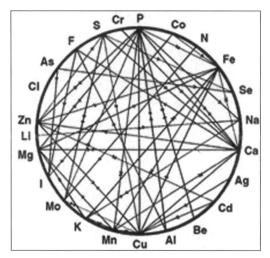

When a single mineral in the body is affected, with either too much or too little, it can have an effect upon at least two other minerals, which will then have an effect on at least two others. It turns out that the field of nutrition can be complex and confusing, and the key to understanding the effects of nutrients is to understand their interrelationships.

In the hair mineral analysis example, we can see the person is low in iron (0.9 mg%) and zinc (11 mg%), and high in copper (4.7 mg%). The mineral wheel can help explain this.

Let's look at copper (Cu), located in the 6 o'clock position on the wheel, to show how complicated treating a zinc or iron deficiency can be. Notice they are connected by a line. It turns out that copper excess negatively affects the zinc (Zn at 9 o'clock) and iron (Fe at 2 o'clock) level by lowering it. Logically, if we are looking at things holistically, if copper is affecting your ability to use zinc and iron, we would want to get rid of the excess copper. Just trying to raise zinc and iron through supplementation wouldn't be the right decision. This is one reason why measuring and not guessing is so important when it comes to your supplement needs.

The next question to ask is what is causing the copper excess? It could be any of the minerals that are in relationship to copper, such as zinc, sulphur, or manganese. If these are low, then copper will be high proportionately. The fix for the iron problem would then be raising these minerals to lower copper, which in turn will raise the iron. Complicated yet fascinating when you know what you are doing. (Farmers have been doing this for generations with their soils.)

There is yet another reason for copper excess, and that is the presence of chemicals and substances that mimic estrogen. This includes things like plastics, pesticides, soy, certain toxic metals, petroleum products, birth control pills, and of course hormones in the food chain. In this example, these estrogens and estrogen mimickers would need to be assessed and dealt with if they were the ultimate reason the person is low in zinc and iron.

What does this mean for you? It means that to flourish physically and mentally you need to get the balance of nutrients and minerals correct. It also means that guessing what to take can be problematic and damaging. The correct balance of nutrients must be maintained and this must be done in a way that measures levels and takes into account the complex interrelationships that exist.

What I find very concerning is that while the vast majority of us recognize the need for supplementation, virtually none of us take the time to figure out what we really need, and as a result play Russian roulette with our health.

Remember that too much or too little of a mineral or vitamin, and the resultant imbalances, are damaging to your health and are what drives the change from normal to abnormal.

Toxic Metals

The second main reason low levels of nutrients like zinc and iron may occur is from the presence of toxic metals. In this day and age, it is extremely unfortunate that toxic metals and chemicals of all sorts have become the problem they are. Some of the more significant are mercury, lead, aluminium, arsenic, and cadmium.

Toxic metals are minerals that do not have any known biological function and are considered poisonous to human life. They are often referred to as heavy metals due to their high atomic weights, and they tend to displace the lighter nutritional metals, such as zinc, calcium, iron, etc. They have become a major cause of birth defects, ADHD, autism, disability, aging, mental illness, divorce, criminality, and all the killer diseases of our day. All toxic metals are extremely acid forming, physically toxic, and neurotoxic.

Toxic metals are present in food, air, and water. In short, they are everywhere and there is no way a person can completely avoid them. Mercury is in our seafood (yes, all seafood), as well as silver amalgam fillings that are usually about 50% mercury. Aluminium is in cans, antiperspirants, municipal water supplies, and in many other common products. Arsenic is in treated wood, drinking water, and many foods. Cadmium was found in McDonald's Shrek drinking cups a couple of years ago in the colored dyes. Children's plastic toys often have cadmium in them, as do many foods due to cadmium being present in NPK fertilizer.

Toxic metals block the ability of your body to use nutrients and they are quite good at it. Mercury's toxicity is such that it will block upwards of 1000 fold of zinc from working properly. Cadmium, aluminium, and copper will also block zinc. Stop and think for a moment what this means. You would need to be consuming 1000 times the recommended amount of zinc just to function normally.

Here is another way to think about the blocking of nutrients. Let's say your cells make an "order" for thyroid hormone. Your body would make the hormone, put it in the blood, and circulate it to the cell that ordered it. Once it arrives it "rings the doorbell" announcing its arrival. Now, picture mercury as the angry doorman. The mercury says to the hormone that the door is locked, that you are fine, and it needs to go away. This is called a channelopathy and is suspected to be one of the most significant reasons for cellular dysfunction and disease. The net result is that your cells are screaming with symptoms but your blood levels are often normal.

Toxic metals also replace preferred minerals. Calcium is the preferred mineral for bone formation; however if calcium is not adequate in the diet, and lead is available, the lead will replace the calcium in the bone. This lead is then serving an actual purpose in the body and is doing a job. The problem is that it is doing the job very poorly and it is weakening the bone, making it more susceptible to osteoporosis and other issues. An analogy is taking a Hyundai fan belt and putting it into a Mercedes. It might work for a short period of time but the Mercedes will be far from optimal in its functioning.

Virtually all of these metals are neurotoxins. They have a tendency to "short-circuit" and otherwise damage the brain and nervous system in many ways, leading to most mental and neurological disorders. The mad hatters of Alice in Wonderland were real. They went mad from using mercury to treat the material they were making hats from.

Contrary to what some believe, you can eliminate toxic metals from the body. However, you must do it in a safe, controlled, and supervised way. Nutritional Balancing accomplishes true elimination and much more. It helps to restore normal functioning of the body, which is the key.

Built into every Nutritional Balancing Program are seven methods that are used simultaneously to eliminate toxic metals. They are:

1. **Improve your energy level.** The elimination of metals is tough work and is impossible without abundant cellular energy.

2. **Provide support for the organs of elimination.** The bowels and kidneys, in particular, must be functioning well to allow for elimination, along with the skin to a lesser extent.

3. **Inhibit the sympathetic nervous system.** The sympathetic nervous system is the state we are in when under stress. This is a breaking down state and it prevents elimination.

4. **Reduce exposure.**

5. **Supplement with heavy-metal antagonists.** For example, zinc lowers copper.

6. **Supplement with natural heavy-metal chelators.** Eating foods with sulphur-containing amino acids (eggs, garlic) aids the body in eliminating.

7. **Other natural detoxification methods.** Near infrared saunas, for example, can help speed up elimination significantly. This is due to the fact that they put your body into the healing parasympathetic state aiding elimination. In addition, when a near infrared sauna causes you to sweat, toxins will leave via perspiration.

The key to eliminating toxic metals and chemicals of all kinds is to enhance energy production, inhibit the sympathetic nervous system, assist the organs of elimination, and reduce exposure to toxins.

The unique value of hair mineral tissue analysis is not just detecting toxic metals but also guiding the balancing of body chemistry to assure their safe and swift removal. When the seven methods are combined, the metals will be removed without the need for synthetic chelators. Toxic metals are often layered deep within body tissues. The recommended diet, supplement, lifestyle, and detoxification program will slowly release these toxins layer after layer. Hidden metals will often be revealed on future mineral tests as they are eliminated through the hair, skin, and other routes.

Putting It All Together

We all want to be healthy and to enjoy everything that life has to offer. With the right information, like that found in this book, and with the right guidance, this is possible. Health is the body's natural state, and where there is a process leading to ill health, there is an opposite process leading to health.

We have established that by the time you can diagnose something, whether it be a lump, growth, x-ray change, blood test, etc., your biochemistry has changed from normal to abnormal. ALL disease, including depression, high blood pressure, increased cholesterol, diabetes, osteoporosis, and osteoarthritis follow this long-established medical fact.

We know that lifestyle stress, whether physical, emotional, or chemical, are the cause of most disease. An interesting aspect to these stressors is that regardless of whether it is physical, emotional, or biochemical, the body reacts in the same fashion by producing the stress hormones adrenaline and cortisol. These stress factors then create the change at the biochemical level, either through nutritional imbalance, excess, deficiency, or toxin.

In Nutritional Balancing, we look to eliminate these stresses when possible. When they can't be fully eliminated, we look to contain them in a holistic way through the use of:

1. Diet

2. Lifestyle

3. Emotional/mental work

4. Chiropractic

5. Correct supplementation

6. Detoxification

Below is a comprehensive example of how a Nutritional Balancing program works with depression. It's important to note that any disease can be viewed in a similar way.

The first step is to identify any physical, chemical, or emotional stresses. This requires time to get to know someone, and to see where emotional or physical issues might lie. Suggestions to eliminate the stress where possible are made. Sometimes it's as simple as getting people to simply slow down.

The identification of chemical stresses requires tests, which is why we need the hair tissue mineral analysis.

In our depression example, serotonin is the "happy chemical." Antidepressants work by blocking the breakdown of serotonin in the brain. Let's stop and look at the process of what is involved in making this hormone, and consider the alternative hypothesis that maybe we just aren't making enough of it, versus the idea that it is breaking down too quickly.

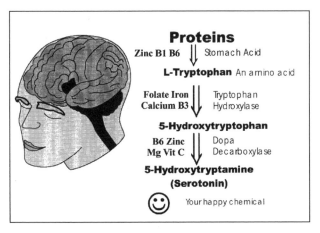

Source - *Visual Textbook of Nutritional Medicine* by Dr. Igor Tabrizian

We start with protein. If you don't eat the protein (turkey with the amino acid tryptophan in it for example), you can't make serotonin. That's the first observation. The next is that to break up the protein, you need proper stomach acid. The number-one selling classification of drugs in the world are for digestion; so it is a safe assumption that MILLIONS have problems here. The next possible problem is that we need zinc, B1, and B6 to even make the stomach acid. Zinc is very deficient in our soils and there is a large percentage of the population (at least 25%) that does not have enough. No zinc, no stomach acid, therefore, no serotonin. Tryptophan is the amino acid you end up with when you break down the protein. Unfortunately, it is the least-abundant amino acid that we get in the diet. Can you see the potential problems here?

Next, to break down tryptophan to 5-hydroxytryptophan, you need adequate amounts of folate, iron, calcium, and B3. If you don't have them, you won't produce the 5-hydroxytryptophan. The same is true for the next step. To produce the serotonin, you need B6, zinc, magnesium and Vitamin C. Notice that zinc is needed again and that you need magnesium, iron, and calcium in these steps.

There is a lot of deficiency in these minerals, isn't there?

The diagram below is a summary chart and you can see all the nutrients we need to make serotonin on the left. As if a lack of vitamins and minerals isn't enough, notice the toxic metals across the top of the chart. In today's toxic environment, they are a huge issue.

Let's use mercury as an example that you may have taken by consuming fish. Even at low levels, the mercury cancels the effect of iron, zinc, selenium, and Vitamin B12 at the cellular level. As we discussed earlier, this means that even IF you have enough zinc in the bloodstream, the mercury will BLOCK the zinc at a ratio of 1000:1. Not good if you want to have healthy normal function.

	Copper block	Cadmium Block	Mercury Block	Arsenic Block	Lead Block	Aluminium Block
Magnesium	X	X				
Iron	X		X		X	
Zinc	X	X	X			X
Calcium					X	
Selenium		X	X	X		X
Vitamin C	X					X
Vitamin B1	X					X
Folic acid	X					
Vitamin B12	X		X		X	

Source - *Visual Textbook of Nutritional Medicine* by Dr. Igor Tabrizian

If a person has nutritional deficiencies, poor stomach acid, or toxic metals in his system, serotonin won't be adequately produced and depression will be present. This also applies to the other brain neurotransmitters required, such as dopamine, gaba, and noradrenalin. Drugs won't fix this, but proper nutrition and detoxification often can. This is basic biochemistry, and very few people are aware of this or have little knowledge on how to use it clinically.

Clearly the use of correct supplements and detoxification are crucial, especially for unwell people. While much of the space allocated to me is focused on this part of the "containment" system, the aspects of emotions, diet, lifestyle, and Chiropractic must not be overlooked. The synergy of all aspects is what actually makes it work, and when you don't address all parameters, you reduce the healing capacity, as there will be more stress on the body than there has to be.

In the hair tissue mineral analysis chart, we can see that our patient is in trouble with her depression. She is showing:

- Deficiencies: Selenium, Zinc, and Iron
- Excess: Calcium and Magnesium
- Imbalance: Calcium/Magnesium, Sodium/Potassium
- Toxins: Mercury, Aluminum and high Copper.

The solution for her depression is quite simple once we have identified these causes.

1. Help her eliminate what stress she can.
2. Incorporate the diet, lifestyle, emotional, Chiropractic, detoxification, and correct supplement components.

I hope it is now clear how stress causes disease, whether it is of a physical, mental, or nutritional nature. As it turns out, our physical, emotional, and chemical well-being are all interlocked. All chronic degenerative diseases can be looked at from a stress and lifestyle perspective, and virtually all can be improved upon. What we often forget is that ALL cells need nutrients (minerals and vitamins) to function properly and ALL cells function better when the levels of toxins are LOW.

To repeat, it doesn't matter what your chronic degenerative disease is, they all follow the same rules.

Conclusion

Nutritional Balancing is a total healing system. When you deal with your stress and properly change your lifestyle to support health, amazing things happen.

When we look at lifestyle-based stress, and specifically and methodically address the deficiencies, excesses, imbalances, and toxins within the body, the reversal of most chronic diseases is possible. Modern medicine is exceptional at emergency care, but has dropped the ball with wellness care.

If you are looking for alternative options to address your health concerns, I suggest you assess your lifestyle, clean up the factors discussed, and get a hair mineral analysis completed to see what is happening with your biochemistry. From this starting point, a comprehensive personalized healing program can be designed for you.

All of our services are available internationally, and we are able to work with you whether you live in Australia, the USA, Canada, or

Europe. For more information, please visit our website at www.life-styleintegration.com.au.

About the Author

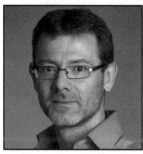

DR. TODD LIZON (BPHE, DC), a renowned educator, is the founder and CEO of Lifestyle Integration. He has been a practicing chiropractor since 1999. He holds a degree in Physical and Health Education from the University of Toronto, and a Doctorate of Chiropractic from the Canadian Memorial Chiropractic College. He has practiced both in Canada and Australia, and currently resides in Far North Queensland with his wife and three daughters.

Lifestyle Integration's revolutionary holistic approach is reshaping the assumptions we hold about how we lose and rebuild health, by ensuring that each and every program we set up is unique to the individual's physical, emotional, and particular chemical needs. We embrace modern technology to assess health through the use of hair tissue mineral analysis, and combine this with the holistic paradigm of health to reverse the disease process.

While we are an Australian-based company, our goal is to improve the quality of life for all, increase active lifespan and productivity, and control or eliminate degenerative disease. We work seamlessly with people from around the world.

We can also be reached by email at:

info@lifestyleintegration.com

CHAPTER TEN
What Is Your Health Potential?

Dr. Jessica Dietrich-Marsh

They told me my daughter would live—it just wasn't the life I wanted for her. I couldn't let it happen. Thus, begins my story...

When my second daughter was six, I found myself in the emergency room thinking she had appendicitis. Her blood work came back with potential leukemia. After several hours and many more blood draws, we had a tentative diagnosis of thalassemia. The next question: was it type A or B? Had any family members died around the age of twenty?

We wouldn't have answers to that death sentence for two weeks.

As we waited on the genetic testing, I read everything I could on thalassemia.

Finally, our appointment at the Oncology Department of Children's Hospital arrived. We walked in prepared for the worst. The doctor walked in almost three hours late, and proceeded to tell us that our daughter was a blend. She had every sign and symptom of thalassemia A but had enough B that she would probably not die early. However, since she was so severe, we needed to be prepared for increased risk of infections, facial deformities, possible height discrepancy, bone deformities, as well as heart and breathing issues. Finally, we needed to be prepared for regular transfusions and the potential removal of her spleen. Furthermore, if and when she married, her spouse would need genetic testing before they had children to rule out the possibility of them having a thalassemia A child.

In one moment, it was as if they had given me back my baby girl (when they removed the death sentence), and then swooped her life away again. I asked how we could help her or prevent any of this, and the doctor sat back, chuckled, and said, "You don't solve this; it's genetic."

He certainly did not give us hope.

Yet I had a knowing that the body renews itself constantly; it is innately programmed to repair and improve. I also knew that I couldn't change my daughter's genetics, but I would somehow find a way to allow those genes to be the best and fullest expression that they could.

In that moment I began my journey into fully discovering the human body. How is blood made? What part of the body must be supported? How do we support it? I discovered that strengthening her bone marrow, kidneys, liver, spleen, and thymus was necessary. I began feeding my daughter a barrage of healthy food and herbal supplements. Within three months, she was the healthiest she had been in a long time. Her improved health continued for years. Then came middle school, when home-packed lunches ended up in the garbage, school lunches became the norm, and the supplements became too much for a busy tween to bother with.

By Christmas of that year, she was down. She was having difficulty breathing and was sleeping sixteen plus hours a day. My beautiful girl, who had overcome so much, couldn't rally herself to go to school, and she developed a cough that was like nothing I had ever heard before. After about a week, I decided to have her blood checked. The blood tests revealed abnormal readings, and it was suggested that she have a transfusion.

On the way to the hospital, I handed her the blood-work results, the books, and all the information I had. I suggested that she review the information and said, "Since you have chosen to be in charge of your own health, you must decide whether you go for a blood transfusion or get back to following the protocol of supplements and food that kept you healthy for so long." This was difficult for me to say, but now was the time for tough love.

As she pored through the information, she came to the realization that she had made bad health choices, and that she was fully responsible for the present state of her ill body. If she was going to be healthy again, she needed to make better choices. Reality hit hard for this young girl. She grew up very quickly that night and said, "Mom, you've done good; I think I'll go back to your way."

For the next few weeks, she took so many herbs and food supplements we lost count. My technique had improved over the years and she was back on her feet and doing great in just two weeks this time. She has maintained her health consistently ever since.

Based on these experiences, I developed a philosophy that includes four core components of health:

- *The importance of good spinal position or structure, which influences the ability of the nervous system to communicate with the body*

- *Living in an environment that is as free of chemicals as possible*
- *Ingestion of proper nutrition, which is the fuel that drives the machine*
- *And possibly the most important: understanding and managing the stress response which monitors your body's functional abilities, nutritional needs, hormone levels, immune system, memories, and belief systems. (I discuss this in greater detail in the emotional section.)*

No matter what health issue patients present with, when proper attention is given to each of these categories, there is no patient who does not experience some level of improvement.

New Ideas

There are four basic steps to learning or accepting a new idea or concept. They are:

Initially, you are unconsciously incompetent *(unaware of one's own environment, existence, sensations, and thoughts; not having the necessary skills to do something successfully)* in your physical health and mental well-being. In other words, it's as if you don't know that you don't know.

It is my hope that by the end of this chapter, you will at least move to the next level and become consciously incompetent *(aware that you do not have the skills to do something successfully, but see there is a problem)*, and have enough tools to move you toward becoming consciously competent *(having an awareness of one's environment, existence, sensations, and thoughts as well as the ability or skills to successfully do something about it)*.

In the last step, unconsciously competent, you master skills, they become second nature to you, and then you are able to teach others. You choose to take personal responsibility for your choices and become masterful.

Identify Yourself

At the time of your birth, you also began to "play the trumpet" of your death. It is inevitable: we all die. What fascinates me is the age at which people decide to accept their fate and roll over, that time when people consciously or unconsciously just quit making great choices. This is a topic I love discussing. At what age did you accept your demise? What are your beliefs around aging? Do you think you will continue to be vibrant and exciting? If not, why not? Have you spent time actively thinking about this subject? What is your vision of you at each decade of life? Do you like what you see? Many times these belief systems, or unconscious scripting, come from the most bizarre places.

A nineteen-year-old once told me that there is no hope for him because his parents had diabetes, so what did it matter? He was confirming his helplessness and also excusing his responsibility for his health. On the complete opposite of the spectrum, I have a ninety-five-year-old patient who is still playing tennis several days a week, driving everywhere, and on absolutely no medications.

What separates the two?

If you haven't thought about it yet, I suggest you take out a notebook and write a description of every decade, from your next birthday to the age you see as your last. To use a great line: failure to plan is a plan to fail at growing older.

It is time to take charge of your life!

Now that you have an idea of your next decades, do you like each stage? If not, why not? What good behavior, that you presently have, can you choose to continue? When do you stop behaviors or start introducing interventions? On what scale do these interventions need to be?

The first intervention I suggest is reviewing your internal scripting. You know, that voice that constantly talks to you. It's the voice that tells you good morning, beautiful or maybe something else not so kind. Where does the majority of this scripting originate? Maybe the TV, or maybe it's the way others have spoken to you.

Many of our preconceived notions come from the commercials running both in and outside of our TV programming. *Programming* is an interesting choice of words, isn't it? Yes, that is exactly what it is—programming the need for drugs, the need for products, the thought processes of demise. The world of advertising is a strong one. Many drug companies now spend almost nineteen times more money on marketing their products than in the research of their solutions.[1]

The more people who take their drugs, the more money they make and the safer they are from financial problems. Multimillion dollar fines for misrepresentation are nothing compared to the billions in profit these companies make. Purdue Pharma was fined Six Hundred Million Dollars for falsifying the research results on the pain drug Oxycontin. For them, it's the cost of doing business—yet people die because of this.

Identify the thoughts that enter your mind by spending a day listening to what runs through your head, and also evaluate the items in your house. Where did the need for these originate? You will find many items are not from family or friends but rather TV. If TV was

1. http://www.huffingtonpost.com/2012/08/09/pharmaceutical-companies-marketing_n_1760380.html

providing the correct information, then we would all be thin, active, and most importantly healthy. Since the outcome is not matching what most would like to achieve, it is time to change messengers.

The next step is to become comfortable with the idea of how wonderfully made your body is. Once you are here, you will begin to realize that most of what is called "disease processes" are simply survival systems that the body takes to ensure it doesn't lose control of whatever it is battling.

This is probably a much different strategy than you have ever encountered. For example, most people have been told that fevers are dangerous, must be immediately treated, and the body temperature must be brought back to normal. Yet, fevers occur for two reasons: to raise the body temperature and burn out whatever virus or bacteria has entered the body; or to pull calcium out of bones and stimulate the white blood cells (part of your immune system). By artificially lowering body temperature with medication, you short-change the body's natural design (or survival system). What you have been told regarding fever is a myth and completely wrong. When you allow the body to function the way it was designed to work, healing occurs.

Emotional States

Stress is now considered the cause of 90% of our diseases.[2] Many people consider work, finances, or marriage as their stress, not realizing that their structure, nutrition, environment, PLUS their emotional stressors are what pile upon the body. Combined, these stressors cause the disease process.

Survival systems are integral in every portion of the human body. They keep the body running and protect you. Your emotional survival systems are no different; you develop conversations with yourself that may or may not be cognitive (at the level of awareness that you pay attention to their message) that in time begin to run your life.

Memories are not created before the age of three,[3] but based on your primary caregiver(s), you become strong in either right- or left-brain thinking. After age three, you begin to put either a logical or an emotional spin on your memories. Each position requires energy and burns through vitamins and minerals differently. Memories and thought processes become even more complicated with the use of antibiotics and the foods that destroy the gut. (I discuss this in detail in the nutritional section.)

Once you begin to tamper with the part of the body that creates the foundation for your emotions, you begin to alter the perceptions

2. http://istpp.org/coalition/index.html
3. http://www.nbcnews.com/health/brain-overload-explains-missing-childhood-memories-6C10070729

of your experiences. Based on those perceptions, you begin to create the script of your life. These are the voices that speak to you; they create your self-worth and self-image. These voices, as well as your life experiences, are also influenced and shaped by the messages your parents, grandparents, friends, teachers, and preachers say to you.

Cortisol, the stress hormone, when released in abundance, can make the brain cortisol resistant. This is similar to the body's tissues becoming insulin resistant for diabetics following too much insulin. When this happens, the mind has difficulty accessing and creating memories. The twist to this is that hormones are created and influenced by your physical structure, environment, and nutrition intake. The more convoluted those items become, the more emotional and/or neurological issues you run up against.

Physical Structure

Most people only look at structure in terms of what it can do for them. Pain is seen as a gauge of its function. If in pain, most people take medications and push through. Traditional uses of pain medications are not without side effects. Did you know that the most common reason for acute liver failure requiring a transplant is the frequent use of Advil or Tylenol?[4]

Advil and Tylenol also significantly increase coronary events. Heart failure is roughly doubled by all NSAIDS (non-steroidal anti-inflammatory drugs), as are upper gastrointestinal complications.[5]

Pain is why many people first visit a chiropractor. They are told we are fantastic doctors for natural pain relief. It's true, we are. In most cases, pain relief is fast and easy. But let's explore some of the other side effects of appropriate Chiropractic care, and the reasons why chiropractors are your best resource for life-long health.

Why Chiropractic is helpful for pain relief can be explained by the anatomy of the human body. The positioning of the twenty-four spinal bones gives protection to the spinal cord, which transmits seventeen trillion messages or decisions every minute. The brain communicates by speeding up the body's processes with messages from the sympathetic, or stress response portion of your nervous system, and slowing things down through the rest response via the parasympathetic nervous system. These two communication styles consistently make minor changes in your body creating homeostasis or perfection. They make up an integral part of your survival system.

The more accurate the position of your spine, the better this system runs. If misalignments are present, then we alter this ability

4. http://www.medpagetoday.com/Psychiatry/Depression/2233
5. http://www.thelancet.com/journals/lancet/article/PIIS0140-6736(13)60900-9/abstract

to function, which activates an alarm that something is wrong. The body then moves into a stress response, causing your system to burn through its hormonal reserves.

For example, when people are under a tremendous amount of stress, they get sick, just as soon as that stress lifts. This is because 90% of the body's vitamin C storage is located in the adrenal glands, which produce the stress hormone cortisol. When under stress, you burn through your vitamin C faster, leaving you susceptible to illness.

The human head weighs ten to twelve pounds and its position is integral to the health of the body. Research shows the weight of a dime, applied to a nerve, is enough to reduce nerve flow by 40 to 60%.[6] This reduction is not necessarily accompanied by pain,[7] since only approximately 10% of your nervous system is made to identify pain.

Falls, trips, minor car accidents, computers, and even texting all slightly alter the head's position on a daily basis. Major injuries to the head from accidents, sports, the birth process, and even a small bang which sets you spinning can dramatically change the speed at which your nervous system fires. This can change how you perceive the world.

Research shows that within six months of a concussion, ADHD or depression are very common symptoms.[8]

Once these misalignments occur and are then reinforced by further injuries, it becomes more difficult for the body to move effortlessly between the rest response and stress portion of the nervous system. We find that the stress response is where most people are stuck.

Let's think of you driving your car with the gas pedal stuck at 50 mph—it's not a big deal if you're on the highway, is it? What would be the result if this happened in a school zone? It's a completely different story; your heart would race, you may sweat, you would worry about what might happen, hopeful that no child crosses the road in front of you, you would try to figure out what to do. Your sympathetic nervous system (stress response) would kick in to send you into reaction mode. Sound familiar?

Chiropractic adjustments help the body relax and move into a more healing state. You can't defend and repair your home at the same time; it takes different tools (hormones, nutrients, minerals). Time must be spent effortlessly shifting between both the stress and rest response.

6. Rydevik, B. L. *The Journal of Manipulative and Physiological Therapeutics.*
7. Hause, M. *Spine.*
8. http://healthland.time.com/2013/01/17/study-reveals-how-concussions-can-trigger-depression/

Environment

Within a minute's time, anything you breathe in or that touches your skin will be present in your bloodstream.[9] Any synthetic chemical will elevate your body's stress response because it is viewed as a poison. Many household items we don't even consider an issue are actually very toxic to the system. To further complicate things, many ingredients are hormone mimickers capable of altering your moods, cycles, and fertility.[10, 11]

For example, lotions often contain urea and parabens. Urea is actually urine, usually animal derived, occasionally created in a lab from chemicals. Paraben is an estrogen mimicker used to plump skin. Its residue is found in many breast cancers.[12]

Most households use bleach-based shower cleaners, plus body washes, and shampoos. While shower cleaners make the walls look great, and body washes smell fantastic, your body is handling a toxic overload with each exposure.

During the shower, hot water opens your pores. Steam excites the cleaner's chemicals as well as the chemicals in water, such as chlorine, and gets them circulating within the shower. With open pores, your body absorbs these chemicals instantly, which moves the body into the stress response. These chemicals can be main triggers for asthma, sinus issues, other breathing disorders, as well as cancers.[13, 14]

EWG.org, a great site for more information, presented a documentary called 10 Americans. It shows that children are now being born with over 200 toxic chemicals in their bloodstream.[15] Again, these chemicals (poisons) force the body to remain in a stress response on a daily basis.

This is one of the easiest of the four categories to conquer quickly and completely on your own. Look closely at the cleaning materials, personal care items, lotions, shampoos, makeup, and other toxic chemicals used in or around your home. Can you pronounce their ingredients? No? Then stay tuned to the last part of this chapter where I give you resources for solutions.

Nutritional Stressors

Most parents quickly learn that certain foods can transform their kids from being gentle and quiet, into something from a horror movie. It was for this reason that I began researching the ingredients

9. http://www.ewg.org/guides/cleaners/content/cleaners_and_health
10. http://www.organicconsumers.org/articles/article_279.cfm
11. http://www.womensvoices.org/wp-content/uploads/2011/11/Dirty-Secrets.pdf
12. http://www.breastcancerfund.org/clear-science/chemicals-glossary/parabens.html
13. http://www.foodrenegade.com/chlorinated-showers-baths-kill-gut-flora/
14. http://www.scientificamerican.com/article.cfm?id=johnson-and-johnson-removes-some-chemicals-from-baby-shampoo-other-products

in the foods that we casually pick up and eat. A great beginning book was *Twinkies Deconstructed*. What I read infuriated me. I began to realize exactly how many toxins are in our foods—and not always properly listed so we can remain informed.

The process of adding preservatives (chemical compounds that mimic the natural vitamins and minerals that have been stripped out of the food, i.e. poisons) was created to make food last longer.[16] However, over time, this noble deed became part of the commodities game upon which large corporations look to increase profits and decrease expenses. One quick way to do that is to decrease the price of your starting materials and eliminate your variables. Organic farming is definitely a variable; so is shelf life. Lab-created food, minerals, and vitamins are cheap, reliable, and stable. Unfortunately they are unrecognized by your body, and most often seen as foreign invaders.

When companies begin to add chemicals in the disguise of fortifying or enriching your foods, food stops being fuel and become just another stressor your body has to deal with. These chemicals are often much more dangerous in children than adults, as the developing brain is five times more sensitive to toxic effects than is the adult brain.[17]

When food is ingested, it goes into the digestive tract, also known as the enteric nervous system. The enteric nervous system is a separate, secondary nervous system consisting of 100 million neurons that can act independently from the brain and the spinal nervous system. If removed from the human body, this system would fully cover two tennis courts. Think of it as a world within your world, containing over 400 known bacterial species (we call them probiotics), which are responsible for breaking down food into the foundation-building blocks for 90% of your brain's chemistry, 80% of your body's immune system, and 100% of your vitamins and nutrients.

Your body's ability to think, feel, move, learn, and repair is 100% dependent on the food you put into your mouth.

The enteric nervous system's ability to function became compromised in 1970 when wheat became a hybrid (two natural plants blended together to make a new plant). Later techniques included exposing the seeds to the industrial chemical sodium azide, which is toxic to the cell's ability to carry oxygen[18] (cellular death leads to cancer) and brain damage (could this be one link to developmental delays and autism)?

---

15. http://www.ewg.org/news/videos/10-americans
16. http://www.livestrong.com/article/413576-the-disadvantages-of-preservatives-in-foods/
17. Blaylock, Russell L., MD. *Excitotoxins: the Taste that Kills.* http://www.blaylockwellnesscenter.com/Literature.html
18. http://www.bt.cdc.gov/agent/sodiumazide/basics/facts.asp

Some scientists will argue that the amounts of sodium azide used are too small to create an issue, but my stance is the body works in nuances not sledge hammers; a small poison over time has the same effect as a large dose at one time. Similarly, the amount of estrogen that the woman makes during her entire lifetime would fit on the back of her thumbnail.[19] Small amounts matter.

Up until 1970, the wheat we used was called Einkorn, the very tall amber waves of grain. It was a high-protein, low-sugar and low-gluten plant.[20] As the hybridization process altered the Einkorn wheat, the small number of gluten proteins turned it into a dwarf wheat plant with twice as many gluten proteins, of which had never before been in our food chain. This also changed the product from a high-protein food source to a high-sugar chemical.[21]

In fact, two slices of whole wheat bread will raise your blood sugar more than two tablespoons of sugar. High-sugar foods increase inflammation, pain, belly fat, strip minerals out of your system, and lead to heart, memory, and immune issues.[22]

Nineteen ninety saw the introduction of a significant change in the government's food pyramid, which now demanded six to eleven servings of grain a day, making the gut virtually unable to repair itself before the next serving is ingested. Think of your gut as a bowling alley with tiny hairs that produce the enzymes necessary to break down and utilize your nutrients. Wheat acts as a bowling ball breaking all of the hairs down with every serving. Often times the "correct bowel function" that occurs after ingestion is actually a "jettison cargo effect" of your body properly eliminating a poison.

With this repeated insult, the gut is very quickly rendered unable to produce B vitamins, the very vitamins that produce energy, help create hormones and neurotransmitters (brain communication materials), and produce blood cells in the bone marrow and nerve sheaths. Lack of B vitamins creates emotional disturbances, irregular heartbeats, insomnia, and manic behaviors.[23]

This alteration within the gut continues to affect the production of dopamine and serotonin without which a greater level of depression, anxiety, mood disorders, and sleep disorders occur.[24] Over time, this will also begin to affect the production of testosterone, estrogen, progesterone (all of your sex hormones) thereby increasing miscarriages and other fertility issues with both males and females.[25]

If that wasn't reason enough to stop eating wheat, when digested it breaks down into exorphins,[26] which are similar to the endorphins

19. http://www.drlam.com/articles/estrogen_dominance.asp
20. http://wholegrainscouncil.org/newsroom/blog/2012/01/research-sheds-light-on-gluten-issues
21. Davis, William MD. *Wheat Belly: Lose the Wheat, Lose the Weight, and Find Your Path Back to Health.*
22. Ibid.
23. http://nutritionresearchcenter.org/healthnews/vitaminbdeficiencies/

(the hormone responsible for the high you receive from exercise, laughter, and lovemaking). Both exorphins and endorphins tell your brain that you are feeling good and you are relaxed. However, exorphins bind to the opioid receptors in the brain addicting you to that high just like heroin does. We know this because when we give binge eaters the same drug heroin addicts get, naloxone, they eat 30% less food.[27]

Just like a drug addict who requires more and more to achieve the same high, you will crave more and more wheat or sugar products to achieve the same sense of well-being. Studies show that eating wheat will cause you to ingest on average an extra 440 calories a day.[28]

When we start to look at what this does during fetal development, we start to see answers to our children's health issues. Research is now showing that the stressors that the father undergoes during his lifetime alter the sperm and affect the cortisol (the body's stress hormone) levels in his children. This means that children can be conceived and already be in the stress response.[29] In utero, the child has no brain blood barrier. Blood brain barriers are designed to keep chemicals out of the brain. This barrier absence means there is nothing that separates the child from everything the mother experiences, such as stress, love, happiness, medications, food choices, food chemicals, sugars, environmental toxins, and drugs from labor.

On top of this, if the mother has not been taught how to address her personal stress response, or if she is in a level of functional adrenal fatigue, she will "borrow" from the fetus's adrenals.[30] This borrowing, plus hormonal mimicking drugs that are commonly used at birth, all can lead to a situation where the infant's adrenals are in deficit at birth, as well as a situation of being addicted to grains and sugars.

If mom continues to ingest wheat while breast-feeding or if formula-feeding (which is made from GMO grains),[31] then these foods will create a poisonous reaction in the intestines that most babies will attempt to throw up. Rather than looking at the issue of why a baby would throw up at birth, many pediatricians simply reclassify this as normal infantile reflux or GERD, and prescribe Prilosec. This drug is only recommended for four to eight weeks of use and

24. Gershon, Michael D., MD. *The Second Brain: A Groundbreaking New Understanding of Nervous Disorders of the Stomach and Intestine.*
25. Smith, Melissa Diane. *Going Against the Grain: How Reducing and Avoiding Grains Can Revitalize Your Health.*
26. http://www.healingmountainpublishing.com/articles/exorphins.html
27. Davis. *Wheat Belly.*
28. Ibid.
29. http://www.newswise.com/articles/view/604192/?sc=dwhr&xy=5031942
30. https://www.inkling.com/read/clinical-gynecologic-endocrinology-infertility-8th/chapter-8/steroid-hormones-in-pregnancy
31. http://www.organicauthority.com/foodie-buzz/eight-reasons-gmos-are-bad-for-you.html

it has NEVER been tested on infants.[32] So, what happens when a child has been using Prilosec for a year or more, a common occurrence when physicians focus on symptomatology instead of searching for the cause? Side effects of this drug include headaches, nausea, diarrhea, constipation, vomiting, blockage of stomach acids needed to absorb and create vitamins (especially vitamin B), and minerals needed for healthy growth patterns. Side effects also include irritability, inconsolable crying, refusal to sleep, changes in the bone marrow which will affect long- and short-term immunity, increased chances of infections, and broken bones.[33]

Once the child is over the age of one, Nexium may be prescribed according to the pharmaceutical manufacturer. The information provided on the package insert suggests use for a short period of time only (eight weeks) with the above common side effects.[34]

Now you have a child who is to small to be on the growth chart , with ear as well as other infections, is a picky eater craving sugar, has increased tantrums, is not napping, and you have parents who are exhausted and with no clue what to do. The short-term outcome is not good, and the long-term outcome is even worse. We see children under age twenty addicted to sugar, markedly obese, and one out of four kids are now diabetic;[35] one out of six are developmentally delayed;[36] one1 in fifty are autistic;[37] and 10% are on antidepressants—and these numbers are growing quickly.[38]

Many studies show that this is the generation that may not outlive their parents due to health-related issues.[39] Research regarding subsequent generations being weaker when nutritional stressors were introduced has been around since the 1930s.[40] Continuing to do the same things your unhealthy parents did, will lead to your children being sicker.

Action Plan

One of the most fascinating metamorphoses I see in the office is how patients' thinking changes when we start working on repairing the gut, balancing the hormones, changing the external environment, and aligning their nervous system. Once the thinking is clear, the hard choices required to improve health become easier.

Fortunately, it only takes about one month of hard work to clean

---

32. propulsid side effects. http://www.rxlist.com/prilosec-side-effects-drug-center.htm
33. Ibid.
34. nexium http://www.purplepill.com/acid-reflux-in-children.aspx
35. http://www.cdc.gov/diabetes/pubs/pdf/ndfs_2011.pdf
36. http://www.cdc.gov/ncbddd/developmentaldisabilities/index.html
37. http://www.nydailynews.com/life-style/
health/50-american-kids-autism-latest-figures-article-1.1302872
38. http://online.wsj.com/article/SB10001424052702303649504577493112618709108.html
39. http://www.nytimes.com/2005/03/17/health/17obese.html?_r=0
40. Pottenger, Francis MD. *Pottenger's Cats.*

up these four areas before we start to see positive changes; some dramatic, but most just enough to say yes to another thirty days of change.

Where do we go from here? First, take a deep breath in and shake it all out. This was a tremendous amount of information that challenges many of your body's perceived survival systems. Which one will be easiest to incorporate? Which ones will be the most difficult? Write them all down. Who will be your advocate for these changes and who will be your naysayers? I will let you decide who you need to talk with the most.

Structural Game Plan

First off, it's important to know that not all chiropractors practice as I do. You must interview your doctors and find out if their mindset and expertise match your health goals. Ask them for the names of five patients who would be willing to speak with you. Talking with satisfied clients is a great practice to utilize when choosing any doctor. If the doctor can't or won't provide you names, is he/she someone you want to have a doctor/patient relationship with? In my office, we encourage testimonials, and always ask patients if they are willing to have us share their success stories.

Getting adjusted regularly allows your body to naturally fluctuate to the survival states it needs in a moment's notice. It keeps your body's communication system fresh.

Movement is also important. Stagnation and sitting is what kills the body the most. Developing an action plan for movement is integral to developing healthy habits and living your full potential.

Simple beginner steps would have you park farthest away from the doors you are planning on entering, and walking. Start slowly and build up your tolerance. Many times, people just rush to the gym to lift weights or run, when their body is exhausted and would have difficulty lifting a fork let alone twenty pounds. Yoga is an excellent first move, as well. It teaches breathing and gentle body movement.

Environmental Game Plan

If I gave you only one website as a reference tool it would be www.EWG.org. They do very well in identifying each section of your life that needs some environmental clean-up. They also have great printouts that list ingredients that are to be avoided, as well as products that do a great job keeping you healthy.

I always recommend starting with cleaning materials, and from there consider the soaps, lotions, makeup, and laundry products. This site is divided into many sections. I suggest that you pick one per month or per week (whichever speed suits you) and change over to better products. Even one major change per month adds up to twelve big ones in a year.

Nutritional Game Plan

It's time to introduce you to real foods. Look at the ingredients, not protein/carb ratios, before you put an item in your grocery cart. If you see ingredients whose names you either can't pronounce or that have more than three syllables, or ingredients you would never be able to purchase at a grocery store, put the item back. Educate yourself on GMO foods and avoid them.[41]

Look at any paleo website and gather recipes. Paleo is a form of eating that eliminates grains, focuses on real foods, meats, vegetables, and good fats. It is one of the easiest eating methods to follow that incorporates all of my nutritional suggestions.

Find people with similar eating habits. I have found that the social part of changing your diet is the hardest. Pick three or four restaurants you can eat at, and when going to parties be prepared to bring your own food. It is ok to be different. If this one is tough for you, spend time journaling your thoughts on food, i.e., what does it mean to you? Once you realize eating is no different than fueling up your car, food will lose its hold over you. Food is fuel for your health. Choose well.

Emotional Game Plan

I have attended almost as many seminars on emotional health as I have on nutrition. Like many of you, my parents were raised by parents who smoked, drank, and not taught to evaluate their emotional needs, let alone the needs of their kids. I have had a blessed life because I chose not to maintain that path. There are a few major players/experiences that shaped how I choose to live my life; and I would like to share those with you.

Tony Robbins' "Unleash your Power" was one of the first classes I ever attended. I walked on fire. Literally. There is not much you can't do after that. This is a three-day event that gave me the inkling that I could change and I could be different. Wow, did it work.[42]

"Lifebook" is a four-day event in Chicago and also available online. My husband and I categorized our life into twelve sections. We identified and wrote down our thoughts and beliefs for each section. It was my first experience with identifying what I had been taught about life and asking if my beliefs aligned with what I wanted to be. Chances are, when you spend some time here, you will find

41. http://www.huffingtonpost.com/margie-kelly/genetically-modified-food_b_2039455.html
42. http://www.tonyrobbins.com/
43. http://www.mylifebook.com/
44. http://bccfreedom.com/

a few subjects that can be rewritten.[43] It is never too late to re-write your future by changing your present beliefs.

If you don't want to travel or attend such courses, get a notebook and spend a day writing down anything that pops into your head— that voice that runs just below your awareness. Write down anything it says to you. These are your body's emotional survival systems; the majority of them are running scripts you are not aware of and will have no desire to repeat. Once you identify statements or beliefs that are not in line with who you want to be, rewrite them one at a time. There is power in putting pen to paper and committing to change.[44]

Finally, if you want personal direction and are interested in a doctor/patient relationship with me, please contact our office. I have put a tremendous team together and we coach all over the world. I would love to be a part of your journey.

About the Author

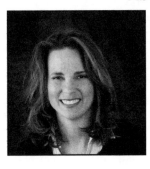

DR. JESSICA DIETRICH-MARSH has been helping patients heal naturally for over eighteen years. Her journey began upon graduation from the Palmer College of Chiropractic in 1994, and the subsequent opening of her practice, Southern Pines Chiropractic Center (now Health Inc.), in Birmingham, Alabama.

It was through her experiences as a mother that Jessica was prompted to expand her practice and knowledge beyond basic structural, Chiropractic care. Her passion for assisting patients to heal naturally, combined with the knowledge garnered from extensive study of the human body, its systems, and the power of Nature, has made her one of the most sought after alternative-health practitioners in Alabama and the southeast.

To date, Jessica has treated over 10,000 patients. Her practice revolves around the belief that healing comes from within and that to achieve your fullest and healthiest potential, you must strike harmony structurally, emotionally, nutritionally, and environmentally.

When she is not seeing patients, Jessica enjoys time on their farm, caring for dogs (one of whom she rehabilitated after it was abused), cats, horses, chickens, sheep, and a bountiful garden . . . Oh, and her beautiful family: an amazing and supportive husband and four strong, healthy, and talented children.

To schedule an appointment, or to book Dr. Dietrich-Marsh to speak at your workplace, church, or civic organization, please visit her website: www.simplerealhealing.com

You may also contact Dr. Dietrich-Marsh at:

Health Inc.
3425 Pelham Parkway
Pelham, Alabama 35124
Phone: (205) 664-7707
Email: Drjessica@simplerealhealing.com

CHAPTER ELEVEN
Begin With the End in Mind

Dr. Krysti Wick

Lost. Look up *lost* in a thesaurus and you will find *missing, gone, vanished,* and *gone astray*. All of those words sufficiently define the majority of my life. Before I discovered the power of Chiropractic, I spent many years wondering where I would end up and how I would get there.

One of my most influential Chiropractic mentors, Dr. David Jackson, often talks about beginning with the end in mind. As you read this book, I expect you have a specific end in mind; most likely, it is a healthy life full of enjoyable experiences with your loved ones.

In my life, it has become abundantly clear that true wellness is a journey and not a destination. Too often people look for the quick fix—I can tell you from personal experience that there is no magic pill, potion, diet, or trick that will create wellness in your life. True health, marked by your body functioning at its highest potential, can only be achieved through continuous effort (regular Chiropractic adjustments, healthy eating, and exercise) and a specific mind-set.

Prior to my awareness of the power of Chiropractic, I spent most of my life believing that I would never be able to change my unhealthy habits. By sharing the personal story of my wellness journey, I hope to inspire you to decide today to change your ending. The single most-important thing that distinguishes us as human beings is our ability to choose; you have the ability to choose health today, no matter what you have believed in the past!

As a little girl growing up in Plymouth, Wisconsin, I told everyone I wanted to be a medical doctor, a pediatrician to be exact. Even then, I knew I would spend my life helping people with their health care needs. I was fascinated by the world of science, and spent countless hours reading about the human body. Every time I visited our family doctor I would tell him about my aspirations to become his colleague one day.

Then, at the age of twelve, I had an accident that changed my life forever. I fell, about fifteen feet, from a barn loft onto a concrete slab. I could not move or walk after the accident, and my dad had to carry me to the car and then to a wheelchair outside of the Emergency Room. The medical doctor told me I had broken a bone in my spine and pointed to the area on the x-ray. All of the other spinal bones were square, while the one I had broken was shaped like a wedge. I was amazed, but in far too much pain to go through my usual scientific questioning with the doctor.

He gave me some painkillers and anti-inflammatory drugs, and told my Dad I would be fine with the assistance of the drugs. The next few weeks were absolutely horrible, as I experienced excruciating pain every single day. The drugs the ER doctor had prescribed not only did not alleviate the pain, but they also made me so drowsy I had trouble staying awake at school. I was a very dedicated student, so this was absolutely unacceptable.

After one exceptionally bad day, my mom decided to take me to the chiropractor. After a few adjustments, I started to feel better. Within a few weeks I was pain free, which was amazing to me! But, even more amazing was the care I received from my chiropractor! At each adjustment, she would ask me how I felt and truly listen to what I had to say. At the age of twelve, this was a big deal. She was compassionate and kind, and made me feel safe under her care.

It was at that point I decided I would become a Doctor of Chiropractic. I knew that if I could help just one person the way I had been helped, it would be worth it.

I spent a few years in high school, and summers while in college, working in my chiropractor's office and observing all the intricacies involved with running a successful Chiropractic Wellness practice.

Fast forward through many years of school and to August 2007, when I graduated from Logan College of Chiropractic. While at Logan, I discovered there are many types of people who enter the Chiropractic profession. Some are interested in sports medicine and the musculoskeletal component of Chiropractic, some are specifically interested in nutritional aspects, and others are looking for a way to contribute to the holistic healing arena. Many people, like me, who have experienced a Chiropractic miracle in their lifetime, feel called to become a chiropractor. This calling, combined with my deep understanding of Chiropractic and the healing potential of the human body, made me certain that this was truly the way I was meant to help people.

Every day as I talk with patients, I help them understand that Chiropractic is based on the premise that the power that made the body heals the body, and true healing occurs from within. Unlike mainstream medicine, which operates under the premise that every symptom requires a drug to reverse it or a surgery to remove the offending anatomical part, the foundation of Chiropractic is removing *subluxations* (misalignments and fixations in the spine) so that they no longer negatively affect the nervous system. Most people have the misconception that chiropractors are focused on bones, when in reality, we are mainly concerned with the nervous system. The health and function of the nervous system is extremely critical as it controls every single physiological function throughout the body.

Chiropractors are especially concerned with the central nervous system, which is housed within the skull and spinal column. Thirty-one pairs of spinal nerves leave the spinal cord through small openings between each vertebra and then travel throughout the body. These spinal nerves are responsible for transmitting impulses from the brain to their respective end organ or tissue. In many cases, spinal vertebrae become misaligned and then fixated (subluxation), which then changes the pattern of nervous system input from those particular nerves. Ongoing and untreated subluxations cause your nervous system to get "stuck in overdrive," forcing your body to remain locked in a constant state of stress.

When your body is stressed due to subluxations, negative information continually travels up through the spinal cord to the brain. The brain then receives that information and perpetuates the stress by sending more negative signals back down the spinal cord, through the spinal nerves to all organs and tissues in the body. This constant stress starts to affect many different areas of your body and a vast array of symptoms can begin to appear. Most patients seek Chiropractic care to relieve their symptoms, and while we are tremendously successful with that, our ultimate goal is to balance your nervous system and restore your body to optimum function. In today's stressful environments, if you are not getting adjusted regularly (weekly or biweekly) to remove subluxations, it is impossible to truly maintain the health of your nervous system.

As adults, we recognize that we experience emotional stress on a regular basis, but are often less aware of the chemical stress (poor diet, chemical additives in many commonly used products, etc.), and physical stress (trauma, poor posture, and work environments) that also cause subluxations. Since your nervous system controls literally every single function in your body, true health and wellness is not attainable as long as subluxations are impeding proper signaling, organization, and flow throughout your nervous system, therefore preventing optimum function.

Despite the fact that I spend most of my days explaining the above concept to my patients, they often find it difficult to grasp because most desire a quick-fix. They think that health is defined as merely being symptom free. When symptoms arise, people seek treatment from their medical doctor; and as soon as the symptom resolves, people assume they are healthy. Very little is done to promote optimum bodily function each day, and the vast majority rely on health insurance to pick up the tab for keeping them "healthy."

For the majority of my life, I was no exception to this mentality. Even though I was adjusted regularly for seventeen years, I did virtually nothing besides that to ensure my body was functioning optimally. It took an extreme trauma in my life to get me to realize that I was lost in the day-to-day existence that consumes most of us, and that I needed to choose a new path in life in order to permanently change my ending.

The beginning of my journey to creating a different path and a new ending occurred on June 1, 2012, when I dramatically discovered that despite the years I had spent studying Chiropractic, I never understood its full potential.

My son, Keaton, was born at 11:37 a.m. on that hot summer day. After a long and difficult labor, Keaton's head became stuck in my pelvis and began to swell. It became necessary for the surgeon to perform an emergency C-section. (I now realize, there are so many things I could have done differently to reduce the stress on my body in order to avoid this ending.) Keaton's head was so engaged in my pelvis that my doctor could not successfully remove him from the C-section incision without the use of a vacuum.

Keaton was not breathing when he was born; he did not cry. Lying on an operating table, staring at the blue sterile drape in front of me as my first child was pulled from my abdomen and hearing no sound was the single most-terrifying moment of my life. I continually asked the doctors and nurses in the room what was wrong and why I did not hear him crying. The look of confusion and anguish on my husband's face was no comfort.

After a few excruciating minutes, the neonatal nurse practitioner came to my side and told me that Keaton was "having trouble breathing," and they were taking him to the Neonatal Intensive Care Unit (NICU). They were planning to use a CPAP (continuous positive airway pressure) machine to force air into his lungs to assist him with his breathing.

I asked to see my son and she told me it would only be for a few seconds. His little face was completely bluish gray and I distinctly remember my heart pounding and my mind racing as I thought about the potential of him never recovering. I was able to give him a quick kiss before the nurse literally ran off with him. I told my husband to follow and not to leave our son's side.

Alone on the operating table, I prayed for my son as the doctor closed up my abdomen and tried to distract me by asking about his name and what we had planned for him when we took him home. Time ticked away, and about thirty minutes later, I was wheeled back into my hospital room, where I was greeted by my mother and sister who had arrived while I was in surgery. I gave them a brief rundown of the events, and burst into tears, asking my sister, "What if he is not ok?" I have never been more scared in my life as I was at the thought of losing my child.

My husband, Joe, entered the room a few minutes later, and joyfully reported that Keaton was breathing with the help of the CPAP machine and the doctors and nurses believed he was out of the woods. I convinced the nurses to wheel my bed down to the NICU so I could finally see my baby. I was not able to hold him due to the CPAP machine, and that, coupled with seeing him with so many wires and devices attached to his little body, was heartbreaking. I was so thankful to the doctors and nurses for saving his life, but deep inside I was so sad that I couldn't adjust him immediately. Prior to going into labor I had already decided our son would be adjusted within an hour of birth; but, just as my plan for a vaginal delivery didn't happen, checking and adjusting him shortly after birth did not come to fruition either.

The following day, the neonatologist examined Keaton, and determined they could now remove the CPAP machine as Keaton's breathing had improved. When the medical team removed all of the straps and tubes, however, it became apparent immediately that something was wrong with Keaton's head. It was completely misshapen and had large lumps and red bruising throughout. The doctors and nurses believed it was something called a subgaleal hemorrhage, something I was not familiar with even with my background, and I immediately asked if they would perform a head CT. The CT needed to be done in order to confirm that the bleeding causing the protrusions was not affecting Keaton's brain.

One of my good friends, a former NICU nurse and now a lactation consultant at the hospital where I delivered, urged me not to Google his potential diagnosis. After the CT results were back and the diagnosis confirmed, I went against her advice and cried as I read that this condition could potentially be fatal. Keaton's neonatologist assured us that Keaton "would be fine," but noted that his head might not look normal for at least six to eight weeks and possibly longer.

My instincts and training told me that Keaton needed to be adjusted immediately, and often. I convinced the NICU nurses to assist me with positioning him so I could check his upper cervical spine (neck). Just as I had suspected, the trauma caused by being stuck in my pelvis and then sucked out with a vacuum had resulted in an extremely severe C1 subluxation. C1 is the very top vertebra in the spine through which the brainstem passes. A subluxation in this area can cause a wide array of extensive problems since it is where communication between the brain and spinal cord begins. I knew that without addressing this subluxation, it would be impossible for Keaton's bleeding to stop and for his healing to begin. I gently adjusted C1 and continued to do so two to three times per day for the next few days. By the time we left the hospital five days later, his head looked completely normal.

In fact, just twelve hours after his first adjustment his head circumference started to decrease and the hematoma (blood accumulation) was visibly much smaller. As a testament to the dramatic change, every NICU nurse commented on how quickly he was recovering. It was during this time of intense personal crisis, when I saw the power of Chiropractic releasing Keaton's Innate healing capacity, that I vowed to take my Chiropractic passion to new levels, as well as change other aspects of my life.

While I have always fully believed that the power that made the body can heal the body, the main weakness in my belief system was the fact that I wasn't living a healthy lifestyle. I have always been extremely self-conscious about my appearance, especially due to the fact that I am a health care provider. I struggled with my weight my entire adult life, and other chiropractors had told me that I would never be successful due to my weight. I am an emotional eater, and used food as my crutch and stress reliever throughout my life.

In 2011, after a Chiropractic seminar, I was fired up and lost fifty-five pounds—only to gain it all back during my pregnancy. After having Keaton, I was tipping the scales at the heaviest I had ever been. I was able to lose some weight in the months following his birth, but the demands and struggles of being a new parent, running a business, and being a successful doctor were extremely stressful. I was not able to return to my pre-pregnancy weight.

In March 2013, I decided it was time to continue the journey I had begun two years before and find my "final answer." My new ending began when I watched the documentary *Doctored* which was widely acclaimed throughout the Chiropractic community. A section of that movie highlighted fellow chiropractor Dr. Anthony Ebel and his wife, Kristina, who shared the story of their son Oliver who was born prematurely and faced a seemingly insurmountable road to recovery. It touched me to watch them describe how they stayed true to their Chiropractic principles throughout their ordeal. While they were eternally grateful to the medical doctors who saved Oliver's life, they allowed the power of the Chiropractic adjustment to turn on Oliver's inborn healing power via the nervous system. The documentary went on to highlight Dr. Tony's practice, one of the largest pediatric practices in the United States, and specifically a case of a boy with autism who was making amazing strides with his communication and behavior due to the Chiropractic care he was receiving at Dr. Tony's office. This section of the documentary brought me to tears, as I knew in that moment that somehow Dr. Tony would participate in helping me change my life. His unwavering commitment to transforming children's lives, by removing subluxations and unleashing the healing power we all hold within our nervous systems, was evident and his conviction was contagious. The difference between the two of us was simple: he was living and breathing Chiropractic every single moment of the day, and I wasn't.

I decided the next step in my journey would be to educate myself further in order to confidently deliver the Chiropractic message with the same level of conviction to each and every one of my patients. While searching for a new approach to delivering the message, I discovered a program called Epic Practice. Created by Dr. David Jackson, a world renowned chiropractor, speaker, and coach, the program consists of online modules focused on communicating Chiropractic in an effective way to every patient. After watching the first few modules, I knew I had found the answer I had been searching for to enhance my communication so my patients could truly hear and feel my conviction. I was one step further on the path toward my new ending, and ready to share my beliefs and knowledge more fully with my patients.

Dr. Jackson phones each new member of Epic Practice to welcome them to the program and provide some personalized coaching. That call led me to admit something to him that I had never admitted out loud to anyone else before. I had known deep down for many years that I subconsciously chose to remain overweight because I used that as an excuse for my mediocrity in Chiropractic. You see, I wasn't fully convicted in my practice and my beliefs. I would often have opportunities to educate patients, friends, and family members about the true Innate healing power of the body—but I would keep quiet for fear of ridicule and rejection. On that call with Dr. Jackson, I admitted to him, after some gentle prodding on his part, that indeed I was choosing to be unhealthy.

The power of admitting that out loud was truly revealing. I urge you to examine the depths of your soul, and if you are struggling with your health, ask yourself why. The answer, if you dig deep enough, may astound you.

Within a month of my conversation with Dr. Jackson, I began to transform myself. The communication in my office dramatically changed, and I saw "light bulbs go on" for so many of my patients. People who were coming to my office for neck and back pain were now getting the big picture and understanding that it was impossible to be truly healthy without being adjusted on a regular basis to restore balance to their nervous system. I began to discuss my own wellness journey with my patients, and took the next step down the path by deciding to commit to eating a healthy paleo diet and exercising regularly.

In that first month, I lost twenty-one pounds. The Universe continued to propel me forward as I discovered that Dr. Jackson had joined forces with Dr. Tony to create a program called Epic Pediatrics. Caring for children has always been the biggest blessing in my practice, and the fact that I could take that passion to a new level by learning from the two doctors who inspired me to start this journey was no coincidence.

In April 2013, the journey continued as I learned that Dr. Jackson would be speaking at the Chiropractic philosophy group I had just joined. Dr. Tony also happened to be a member of this group as our practices are only two hours apart; so I had had the opportunity to meet him briefly and tell him I was committed to the Epic Pediatrics program. On April 22, 2013, I had the pleasure of meeting Dr. Jackson in person and sharing my transformation with him. I sat through his ninety-minute presentation with tears in my eyes; once again thanking God for placing him and Dr. Tony in my life. I could tell in that moment that I had changed forever and there was no going back. I had finally chosen health and wellness; I had decided that I would live life to the fullest and lead the way so that I could truly help my patients.

Each and every day the choice I have made to live a healthy lifestyle is a struggle; but I can tell you that it does get easier. The most important thing is to choose to remain true to your mind-set and remember that eating healthy, exercise, and getting adjusted on a regular basis will continue to erase all of your prior bad habits. The pure joy that comes with your body functioning on an entirely different level will also help to propel you forward.

Typically choosing to begin the process of change is the most difficult for people who struggle with their health. In many cases, they feel so overwhelmed by their symptoms or state of dis-ease that they never find the motivation to start heading in the other direction. In my life, the starting point was mental. I suffered through a great deal of personal trauma and stress which made me re-evaluate my health, my passion, and every single one of my choices—and I finally admitted the impediment that was my biggest obstacle.

I urge you to begin by working hard to uncover your personal obstacle that is subconsciously keeping you from a healthy mind-set. On a daily basis, I listen to patients who are convinced they will never regain their health. In general, if they truly believe that, they will probably be correct. The mind is powerful; negative thinking perpetuates stress, which has a profoundly negative impact on your nervous system.

As already stated, *true health* is defined as optimum function and that is impossible unless your nervous system is completely balanced so it can combat your daily stressors. Uncovering your crutch is going to be painful and it is going to take an extraordinary amount of honesty on your part; however, once you have identified the problem and admitted it out loud, your wellness journey can finally begin.

To aid you in your journey, I would like to highlight three important things you need to conquer on your road to wellness: chemical, physical, and emotional stress. These three culprits are responsible for creating subluxation patterns that lock your entire nervous system into stress mode which perpetuates your state of ill health. Let's examine each area and look at options to overcome these stressors, as you embark on a journey to your new, healthy lifestyle. It is important to note that these are generalized suggestions and your personal chiropractor will be able to assist you in formulating more personalized approaches to improving each area of stress.

Physical Stress

Get adjusted regularly. Regular Chiropractic care is paramount when it comes to your wellness journey. Virtually every other suggestion I make will have a much lesser impact if your nervous system is not free of interference from subluxations.

Get moving. Regular exercise is vitally important to minimize physical stress on your body. Sedentary lifestyles, desk jobs, electronics, and poor posture have created an extraordinary amount of stress on your musculoskeletal system.

Chemical Stress

Clean up your diet. I encourage you to begin Paleo eating, as I have, to ensure that the chemicals and additives that permeate the standard American diet do not have an ill effect on your health. The Paleolithic diet consists of mainly wild fish; grass-fed, pasture-raised meats; eggs; vegetables; fruit; fungi; roots; and nuts. It excludes grains, legumes, dairy products, refined salt, sugar, and processed oils. I often call this an "anti-inflammatory" diet since the foods that are excluded perpetuate inflammation in the body. Severely limiting or eliminating these foods is extremely important to regain and maintain optimum body function.

Use natural household products! Many household cleaners and hygiene products contain extremely harsh chemicals which contribute to the chemical stress level in your body. Whenever possible, search for natural alternatives. In my home, for example, we commonly use vinegar as a cleaner. Natural soaps, shampoo, deodorant, and toothpaste are also essential. Babies and children especially are susceptible to the toxicity of the chemicals in these products; so make sure you are choosing natural products for the littlest members of your family.

Emotional Stress

Get a massage. I have found that patients who receive regular massage therapy typically have a much healthier emotional state. Not only is massage extremely helpful for your muscular system, it allows you some meditation time which assists with combating any emotional stress. I often recommend weekly massages to my patients with severe stress and gradually reduce the frequency to monthly as their stress levels decrease.

Discover your strategy. Regular exercise, counseling, and journaling are other effective ways my patients manage their emotional stress. Typically, this is a difficult area to eliminate for most adults and it will take time for you to find a coping strategy that works well for you. Once you feel your stress level is decreasing, make sure that you document the process you used to achieve that goal. In today's society, stress is constant and it is very important to establish healthy habits to continually deal with it.

These are just a few of many strategies designed to decrease stress levels. As you begin to live these strategies, I'd like to encourage you to consider expanding that use to your entire family. We often don't think about our children experiencing stress, however, most subluxation patterns begin in children prior to birth due to stress throughout pregnancy. Birth trauma, everyday falls, poor diet, vaccinations, and harsh chemicals all contribute to stress on their tiny bodies on a daily basis.

Remember, without balancing their nervous system and

eliminating the stress that caused your child's body to reach a state of ill health, no prescription, surgery, or other remedy will allow their body to return to optimum function. Imagine what Keaton's ending could have been if I had not started adjusting him as soon as possible. His head condition could have worsened and caused a host of additional problems. Allergies, asthma, colic, ADHD, autism, bed wetting, sensory processing disorder, and so many other childhood diagnoses are deeply rooted in the nervous system. Any child suffering from such symptoms could potentially have a life free of these debilitating conditions if a pediatric chiropractor would have adjusted them as newborns.

Every child deserves to live a healthy life, free of nervous-system interference, so they can express their full potential. The best gift you can give your children is to have them checked for subluxations and adjusted as needed on a weekly or biweekly basis for the rest of their lives. My new ending contains a burning desire to educate as many parents as possible about the power of removing nervous-system interference from their child's body.

And remember, it's never too late to get checked for subluxation.

As you can tell, I no longer feel lost. I have found my specific end, a healthy life and a renewed passion for my chosen field of Chiropractic. As I checked the definition of *found*, "to build or establish the foundation or basis of," I realize that my journey has led me to build a strong foundation for helping people, and that is just what Chiropractic does. I wake up and thank God every day that I can go to work and affect someone's life in a positive way. What is more, since my awakening, I have realized, without a shadow of a doubt, people's lives are at stake. Every day new patients walk into my office with a lengthy list of medications and I can see in their eyes how it affects every facet of their beings. I am on a mission to educate them about their own Innate healing power and share my story so they know they are not alone.

I urge you to find a chiropractor who will take the time to listen to you and get to know you on a deep level. It is critical to find someone who will not only educate you about healthy lifestyle choices but also provide support and understanding.

What will motivate you to change your ending?

The purpose of sharing my story is simple: I have faced a trauma so great that it inspired me to change my life. Change is possible without trauma as long as you have the mental fortitude to make it happen. If you are feeling lost, missing, gone, vanished and gone astray, do what is necessary to **find yourself**!

Your health and happiness, and that of your family, depend on it!

About the Author

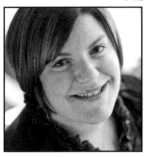

DR. KRYSTI WICK has owned and operated River Shores Chiropractic in West Bend, Wisconsin, since December 2007. Chiropractor, wife, community leader, and devoted mother, she lives in the country just north of West Bend with her family and their three dogs.

Her present and past local board member involvement includes roles with the Volunteer Center of Washington County, Citizen Advocates, Kewaskum Chamber of Commerce, West Bend Chamber of Commerce Leadership program, Rising Professionals on the Move, and the Enchantment in the Park Steering Committee. Always seeking a means to encourage others pursuing careers in health care, she has held positions as an instructor at the University of Wisconsin-Washington County, Blue Sky School of Massage Therapy, and Moraine Park Technical College. Professionally, Dr. Wick is a member of the American Chiropractic Association, International Chiropractic Pediatric Association, Wisconsin Chiropractic Association, and the Chiropractic Society of Wisconsin.

She is dedicated to providing effective Chiropractic care that is tailored to meet the needs of each individual patient. While especially enjoying the pediatric aspect of her practice, she offers care for the entire family—infants to grandparents. She is available for speaking engagements on a variety of health-related topics. For more information, please visit her website: www.rivershoresChiropractic.com

You may also contact Dr. Krysti Wick at:

River Shores Chiropractic
705 Village Green Way, Suite 105
West Bend, WI 53090
Phone: (262) 334-4070
Email: info@rivershoresChiropractic.com

"Chiropractors do not treat diseases,
they adjust the wrong
which creates disease."

B. J. PALMER, DC, THE SCIENCE OF CHIROPRACTIC, 1920

CHAPTER TWELVE

The Intricate and Delicate Power of Self

Dr. Larisa Shevchuk

I am going to re-introduce you to you—the intricate and delicate, yet powerful, you. Your body is a thousand times more amazing than an exquisite mechanical watch that is controlled by tiny mechanisms working in unison. Similar to how a watch needs winding up, you might need a tune-up to your inner working system too.

I am a nervous system and spine specialist. I help people be their best by having their nervous systems function well. In turn, they get to be self-expressed in the world and contribute fully. When humans are functioning well and are joyous, everything is possible in the world.

This is the story of how I became a health care provider.

I served as a Registered Nurse for seven years, walking with my patients on the fine line between life and death every shift I worked. It is four in the morning, and I am working a night shift at St. Paul's Hospital in the Intensive Care Unit. I watch the monitor that records the electrical impulses of the beating heart and maps out the rhythm for me to read. My patient is hooked up on life support and tubes are entering and exiting every crevice of his swollen body. My patient is unconscious and has been like that for the last five weeks. He relies on medical technology to have every breath blown into his lungs and a medical drip for his heart to beat, along with other concoctions of drugs to sustain his life. Nurses turn him every two hours and his body is starting to break down from not moving. He is losing up to five percent of his muscle mass every day. If he makes it out of Intensive Care, he will have to re-learn how to walk and his digestion system will have to learn how to work again.

Despite the hard work as a nurse, there was joy and happiness as well. The strength of a human spirit to survive the toughest ordeal, a smile in the toughest moment, inspired and amazed me. Miracles happened. A patient we never expected to pull through survived and healed well enough to come back a year later to thank the nurses. A team of nurses and doctors working in unison during a code blue, barely saying a word to each other, yet all knowing what to do and not getting into each other's way, just like a well-rehearsed play.

We were amazing at emergency situations—but what we weren't good at was promoting good health and preventing ill health. Prevention in the hospital world consisted of early intervention, starting people on medications, or sending them for biopsies. The idea was to catch the disease sooner in order to change its course.

The first response is always medication, then see what happens. If one medication didn't work, then we tried another, or a combination of a few. If people experienced side effects, we had a medication for that too. Many times doctors weren't sure what antibiotic to prescribe, and we would try several before we would get control of an infection. Same with heart medications—there were a few "go-to" medications that most people received, and if it didn't work, we tried another. (The latest research on these medications was often presented during fancy dinners or nice wine-and-cheese events.)

It was common to hear people cough on the Cardiac Unit because it is a side effect of a common blood-pressure medication, Ramipril. In the few years I worked in the hospital, I administered medications that have since been deemed dangerous and pulled off the market.

My morning shifts on the Cardiac Unit always started with me looking into every room to quickly check on my patients to see if they were okay. My next ritual was dispensing their morning medications, which ranged anywhere from four to ten pills just at breakfast time. At times like that, I wondered, "How did I end up being a dispensary of pharmaceuticals to keep people 'healthy?'"

My initial goal was to become a medical doctor. I am glad now that my parents couldn't afford to put me through medical school. Because of that, I chose to become a nurse first, and then later I would put myself through medical school while I worked as a nurse. As I started my nursing career, I questioned more and more if I ever wanted to be a doctor. The human body, that I respected so much, was treated as a sum of parts. The body was seen as weak and failing, and technology and drugs were there to save it.

It just didn't feel right.

The miracles were written off as something unexplainable. I remember a time when a doctor couldn't find a suitable vein on a failing patient right after surgery and the whole team was whirling around the person, shouting orders and pulling her out of the grips of death. She was fully awake and so scared—she didn't say a word but her eyes said it all. I knew she thought she would die right there in the midst of the scuffling and rushing of hands to remove her gown to attach monitors and to manage her bleeding incision. She would die while everyone paid attention to her alarming monitor and drips, and no one paid attention to her being so scared she couldn't even take a breath. I looked at this woman and connected with her as a human being, not a combination of numbers, alarms, fluids, and oozing blood. A sense of peace came over me and I knew it was up to me to keep her calm. All I could do was "be in the moment" for her and ask her to stay calm.

I explained what we were doing. I held her hand and talked into her ear, encouraging her to take a deep breath and to relax. I let her know that she was in the right place at the right time and that everyone knew what they were doing. We were experts doing everything to make sure she was okay. I told her to relax, and said, "I will stay with you the whole time and you will pull through." I talked loud enough for everyone to hear, and as I talked, everyone calmed down and stopped hurrying over her. Their arms started to move in unison and with grace. Everyone believed she would pull through, as I reassured her. And she did. Her vitals stabilized, the bleeding stopped, and I knew that my calm presence and reassurance played a big role. I never knew myself to be that powerful and in tune with another human being. I am very clear that if I wasn't present that day, despite my being scared too, the woman might have died. My colleagues worked in desperation, they followed the motions, and in their minds they knew the outcome.

In that experience, I recognized that I respected the power within a human body, and the value of being connected to another human being like never before.

As a junior nurse, I would have never had the courage to talk to my patient like that. I would have never permitted myself to connect with another human being like that. In emergency situations, I would have looked for the reassurance from the doctors, for I believed they knew what to do.

With years of experience, I learned that medical professionals often didn't know what to do and it was sometimes a guessing game of interventions, medications, and surgeries. Hospital work ate away at my soul; the constant struggle, death, and misery overshadowed the joy of healing that did happen.

Seven years later, I realized I was part of *sick care* and not *health care* as I had dreamed. I watched thousands of dollars being spent in one day in intensive care that saved people's lives but didn't make them any healthier.

Working shift work and flipping from days to nights, I needed help to recover. I utilized over-the-counter medications to help me sleep during the day to have me ready for the night shift. What I found worked best was not medication but regular exercise and meditation. Meditation was the best way to take care of my mind while it was racing with the events from work and preventing me from sleeping. I knew that I couldn't spend another thirty years working as a nurse and a different career was eminent. I also knew I no longer wanted to be a medical doctor.

I had been under Chiropractic care since the age of twenty. I always liked natural healing and it made sense to me to see a chiropractor for minor aches and pain rather then popping a painkiller. When I was evaluating what to do next, it just clicked. Chiropractic was it! It was everything that I was fascinated about—the amazing human body.

The cluster of living cells working together, growing, healing cuts and bruises, mending bones, and creating scars—its own universe of intelligence inside. Just like the rain, lakes, and ecosystems of the world working together, the human body has its own universe inside, every part working harmoniously together. We started from two cells and grew into complex billions of cells, each knowing what was needed to keep us alive and thriving.

The answer was clear to me and I packed my bags and moved across the country to attend the only English Chiropractic school in Canada—Canadian Memorial Chiropractic College. My family and friends held an intervention for me. They sat me down and added up how much this adventure would cost me: four years of lost income, loans to cover student fees, plus the cost of living, and relocation. It came to over half a million dollars. My friends urged me to stay in Vancouver and start a business, if I really wanted to leave nursing that bad. My parents urged me to get married to my fiancé and have a baby, if I wanted something new and different. My mom pleaded and was worried that my engagement would not survive this new adventure. Something in my heart told me it was the right thing to do. My fiancé, now my husband, was the only one who supported me. (Interestingly, my husband and I were the only ones in our circle of family and friends who were under regular Chiropractic care at the time.)

We knew there was something special about Chiropractic. I knew that I was destined for something special in this life and working with Innate Intelligence of the body through Chiropractic was it. (Since then, my family has started Chiropractic care and they are amazed with how well they are feeling and how much their health has improved. My parents started to dance tango and recently came back from a special dancing trip in Argentina, where they danced tango every single night. They continue to dance weekly.)

I spent the next four years learning the marvels of the human body and how we, as chiropractors, support the body's inner workings to work well by having a healthy nervous system. I knew each day spent studying was worth it. I knew I would be saving lives again and be part of health care. I was excited to be supporting the body working well as a whole, naturally, and not by its parts.

By having the body work as it was designed, and people not being alerted that something is not working by headaches, neck and back pain, shoulder and foot pain; they can concentrate on who they are and what they are meant to do in life, and make their difference in the world. When everything in your body works and your health is well you get to be the most creative, most loving, most gracious, most contributing human being. You are a joy to be around.

I felt I owed it to humanity to provide a service that allowed people's bodies to work well. I knew something that made the human frame function as it was divinely designed by keeping the nervous system free of interference.

What chiropractors do can be explained by sharing insights about a children's game. Remember a game we played as kids, joining hands in pairs and standing to form a tunnel, then each pair taking a turn and running underneath the arch of joined hands? Imagine that is your spine. It protects and supports your spinal cord, it is the lifeline that connects your brain to the rest of your body. It's the computer system that operates, controls, and receives all the information about your body and in turn adapts to your environment.

Your body shivers when it's cold to warm up, and sweats when it's hot to cool down. Your heart beats faster and stronger when you are running and the blood rushes to your muscles. You don't have to tell your body to do so, your body is intelligent and it responds to the stimuli and the environment around you by sending messages via your nervous system. Your brain and nervous system receive the information of where you are in space and regulate how fast your heart must beat. It monitors where to rush the blood—to muscles so you can dance, to your vocal cords so you can sing, or to your digestive tract so you can digest and absorb the essential nutrients. Your brain comes up with innovative ideas that have never been thought before. Your brain experiences love and joy, sorrow, and sadness. The power of your mind is so strong that even your thoughts can change your physiology.

If you think of biting into a ripe sour lemon, your mouth will salivate. When you think of a happy moment in your life, you experience joy and smile. When you think of a tragic moment, your throat tightens and tears swell up in your eyes. Those things are not happening to you right now, yet the mere thought of these events creates the physical changes in your body.

Remember those kids that linked hands and formed a tunnel and had other kids running under their linked hands? Imagine that one pair of kids shifted into the tunnel. It would be challenging for the kids to run smoothly through the tunnel, they would get stuck and have to get through the misaligned kids. The kids represent the vertebrae that surround your spinal cord. The kids running through the tunnel are the nerve impulses travelling from your brain to your body and back. It would be more challenging for the messages to get through where they were going if interference was created. The speed at which electrical impulses travel through the nerves ranges from 4 m/sec and up to 120 m/sec (432 km/hr) depending on the type of the nerves.

A vertebra in the spine that is restricted and not moving within its normal range is referred to as a *subluxation*. The subluxated joint will have an impact on the nervous system and the nerve that exits between two vertebrae in your spine. In addition, your body will need to expand extra energy to deal with the rogue joint by creating inflammation in the area, because that is how the body heals itself. Your intelligent body will rush extra blood to the area with much-needed extra nutrients, oxygen, and helper cells to clean up the area and repair the tissue. The surrounding muscles will be in spasm to protect the area. The ligaments and tendons around it will also be affected, sending pain signals to your brain. Your body is signaling that something is in need of attention. Your body will work hard to repair the slight injury and to restore proper motion.

While you sleep, your body is in repair mode. Its internal signals search the body for mild wear and tear to repair. That is why sound and consistent sleep is so important. It is your body's repair mechanism.

This is also why eating nutritious foods that nourish and repair your body is important. Whole unprocessed foods nourish your body, while providing you with energy and vitality. Processed, fried, and sugary foods give you instant energy but not sustainable energy that can be used to repair the body. Moreover, those foods are actually inflammatory in nature, thus making your body work harder to detoxify your body of those foods laden with chemicals. Foods that are full of ingredients that you cannot pronounce inflame your gut, your joints, and the lining of your blood vessels. The joints get achy and swollen, and wear out faster than your body can repair them.

There are plenty of commercials on TV to sell you painkillers that claim to help you with pain and dysfunction. Yet we know that drugs don't fix the problem, they simply mask the symptoms. When the digestion system gets upset, they propose the use of that plastic pink remedy called Pepto-Bismol or other anti-heartburn medications. This too simply masks the symptoms and doesn't help you be healthier.

Blood vessels get inflamed and raw, making fat and plaque easy to stick to their lining, something that does not happen on the smooth, shiny surface of a healthy blood vessel. The common cure today, to avoid heart and vessel disease, is to give people anti-cholesterol medication to reduce the amount of fatty substance (cholesterol) and thus have less chance of it sticking to the vessels. I noticed a trend of people as young as thirty being put on these medications (Simvastatin and similar drugs). Those people will be taking these medications for the rest of their lives. Those medications are robbing the body of the cholesterol that is needed to make up every cell membrane in the body and the cholesterol essential for the production of all hormones and vitamin D. These medications also rob the heart muscle of coenzyme Q10 which is needed for the heart muscle to beat strong and stay healthy.

Many people also get back pain as a result of these medications, a very common side effect. Would it not be logical to stop eating foods that are inflammatory in nature and support the body by having good nutritious foods? Would not it be logical to keep the heart and blood vessels healthy by going for a thirty-minute walk every day?

Our body is a self-contained universe. A cut is repaired by blood delivering platelets that stop the bleeding and bring cells to repair the injury. A broken bone is mended by growing new bone. An infection is taken care of by increasing your body temperature (creating a fever) to burn off the bacteria or virus.

Supporting the natural way of life just makes sense, allowing for the body to do what it is designed to do best: maintain its own ecosystem. Supporting the immune system to be healthy and strong makes sense rather than taking a drug that dries out the mucus while fighting a cold, or suppressing the coughing mechanism in our brain while the lining in our lungs fight off the infection inside. It is crazy to take drugs to suppress these natural occurrences. These drugs might make us feel better instantly, but the cold can last up to two weeks longer than if the natural processes were allowed to run their course and the body was supported with plenty of fluids, rest, and vitamin C. The chicken soup moms used to feed their kids when they were expressing symptoms, and then tucking them into bed for rest and repair, was the best way to go!

What does all of this have to do with Chiropractic? Chiropractors view the human body as a whole, intelligent organism that knows exactly what it is doing. Chiropractors check your spine to ensure the joints are moving well and thus the electrical impulses are travelling uninterrupted to and from the brain for your body to communicate properly. We live in a fast-paced society and are conditioned to seek quick relief and gratification. We see ads on TV every day promoting painkillers to stop a headache, or pain in our hands. However, a painkiller simply masks the symptoms and does not help address the solution. Painkillers and anti-inflammatory drugs actually prevent the body from doing its work of protecting and healing injured areas. These drugs decrease the normal inflammatory response and reduce your body's ability to feel the pain; thus moving the injured area and preventing proper healing.

You might ask, "If the body is self-healing and self-regulating, then why would I need a chiropractor to have my spine checked?" In a perfect world, your body could probably heal itself without any intervention. However, we live in the world of constant sitting, little physical activity, and a lot of stress. The majority of people eat less than nutritious foods at best and foods with no nutritional value at worst. The simple answer is: you have a spine. Everyone needs a highly functioning spine and nervous system for healing and repair. That's why regular Chiropractic checkups are a must. Just like having a dentist check your teeth regularly, your chiropractor checks the joints of the twenty-four bones in your spine to make sure they are moving well and the nervous system is functioning at its best. And, just like dentists recommend you take care of your teeth at home by brushing, flossing, and eating well, chiropractors have their recommendations to take care of your spine by doing stretches and exercises for your back and overall well-being.

In addition, to experience your best health, your chiropractor might talk to you about nutrition and supplements, sleep hygiene, exercise, and teach you to think well. Our goal is to support you in reaching your best health possible by supporting your body's natural processes. Achieving optimum health is a partnership between you and your chiropractor.

In my office, I use the mnemonic DREAM to teach my clients five aspects of good health. D stands for Diet, R for rest, E for exercise, A for proper alignment, and M for mind. I focus mainly on the spine and nervous system function by checking and restoring motion to the joints in the spine. This is accomplished by delivering a gentle manipulation to affected joints. At times, it might be necessary to check other joints, such as shoulder, elbow, wrist, hip, knee, and feet to make sure they are moving well. While your spine is healing, your chiropractor will be checking your spine and adjusting it if needed. Other joints that may require adjusting to help the brain receive proper information from the joints will also be considered.

At first you might need to come in more often as change is introduced to your body. How often you come in for an adjustment will depend on how long you have had the injury and the state of your overall health. These issues determine how long the healing will take. I compare Chiropractic care to painting a wall: it needs to be done in thin layers and given time in between to dry.

Chiropractic creates small changes that the body needs time to accept and re-learn. At first, your spine will require more adjustments as it tends to return to its misaligned state. With time, though, your body will begin "holding" adjustments better and may only require periodic checkups and tune-ups.

I am a human and animal chiropractor. I ensure the nervous system is functioning well in babies and adults and pets. If you and your family are looking to have a natural solution to your health, book a checkup with your local chiropractor or call our office. I will be happy to take care of you, your family, and your pets. I love what I do and everyone I interact with. I proudly live by the quote:

> "The only way to be truly satisfied is to do what you believe is great work. And the only way to do great work is to love what you do. "
>
> STEVE JOBS

About the Author

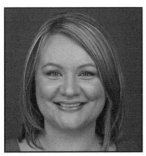

DR. LARISA SHEVCHUK has been a health care provider for over ten years. She first worked as Registered Nurse in Vancouver, British Columbia, for seven years. The body's natural ability to heal inspired Dr. Larisa to become a chiropractor. She ensures that her clients' spines and joints are moving well and their nervous systems functioning well.

Dr. Larisa is helping people and animals in Toronto, Ontario, to be their healthy best by working with the body's Innate ability to heal.

To make a health appointment for you and your family, or to book Dr. Shevchuk to speak at your workplace, church, or civic club, please visit her website: www.sheismychiropractor.com

You may also contact her at:

Total Health Chiropractic Centre
3555 Don Mills Road, Suite 200
Toronto, Ontario M2H 3N3
Office: (416) 492-6563
Direct: (416) 898-2670